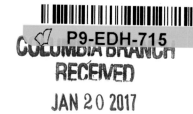

Living Better with Hearing Loss

A Guide to Health, Happiness, Love, Sex, Work, Friends . . . and Hearing Aids

KATHERINE BOUTON

WORKMAN PUBLISHING • NEW YORK

Library of Congress Cataloging-in-Publication Data is available.

eISBN 978-0-7611-8508-6
Print ISBN 978-0-7611-8722-6

Design by Janet Vicario

Workman books are available at special discounts when purchased in bulk for premiums and sales promotions as well as for fund-raising or educational use. Special editions or book excerpts can also be created to specification. For details, contact the Special Sales Director at the address below, or send an email to specialmarkets@workman.com.

Workman Publishing Company, Inc.
225 Varick Street
New York, New York 10014-4381
workman.com

WORKMAN is a registered trademark of Workman Publishing Co., Inc.

Printed in the United States of America

First printing May 2015

CONTENTS

INTRODUCTION

I had no idea it was possible for a thirty-year-old to lose most of the hearing in one ear overnight without any apparent explanation. But it happened to me. Back then, I didn't have an internist, much less an ear, nose, and throat (ENT) specialist. I certainly didn't know how to find an audiologist. Hearing aids were for old people, and anyway they didn't work.

Within a few years, the left ear loss had worsened and was joined by progressive loss in the right ear. Still, I stumbled through life, increasingly deafer with every year. By the time I got hearing aids twenty years later, I was seriously hard of hearing. And it took me another decade before I admitted to myself and finally to others that I had a disability, and that I needed help.

This is what my hearing loss feels like—even with a cochlear implant and hearing aid:

SCENARIO #1

My husband sneezes in the next room.

"What?" I say.

Mumble mumble.

"What?"

I get up and go to the door of his office. "*What* did you say?" I ask impatiently.

He looks up from his computer. "I didn't say anything."

"Then what was that big loud noise?"

"I was just sneezing."

SCENARIO #2

The phone rings.

Ever optimistic—or perhaps, ever in denial—I pick it up.

"Hello?"

"Hi, Mom. It's Will."

"You want to talk to Will?"

"No, it *is* Will."

"Will? He's not here."

"No, it is Will!"

"Can you text me?"

It's only when I get the text that I realize I've been talking to my son.

SCENARIO #3

Someone on the street calls, "Taxi!"

I turn around.

"Taxi" sounds like "Katherine!" to me.

Unfortunately, as these examples show, my hearing is far from perfect—not to mention far from normal, even with the hearing aid in my right ear and the cochlear implant in my left. In general, the best technology can restore hearing only partially when the loss is as severe as mine. This is something that people with normal hearing don't understand. Sometimes even audiologists don't understand it. Certainly, anyone getting a hearing aid for the first time expects that it will correct the hearing loss. Glasses work. Why shouldn't a hearing aid?

The mishaps described above are relatively harmless. My family is forgiving. But when I worked in a high-pressure job at *The New York Times*, the stakes were much higher. I never made a major error, but I was not an optimal colleague. Most of my coworkers didn't know I had hearing loss, and those who did had no idea how serious it was. But what they did know—when I failed to answer a question, or when I failed to respond to something they'd said, or when I asked a question that someone else had just asked, or made a comment that someone else had just made—was that something was off.

I was either a snob or stupid or aloof or bored or burned out.

I thought I'd fooled my boss, too, and I had. His impression was that I was not a team player, and he pushed me out of my job.

Why We Ignore Hearing Loss

Most hearing loss comes on slowly, usually from noise exposure or aging. People may not even know they have a problem, because hearing tests are not routinely given at annual physicals. They may feel confused, and not notice missing certain sounds. It's easy to forget that the wind blowing in the trees is a sound, and not just a sight. Water running in the sink makes noise.

They can't hear in a noisy place, but they blame the place—this restaurant is too loud. Or they blame the speaker—she mumbles, he has a mustache, a foreign accent, thin lips. It doesn't occur to them that the problem may be theirs, not someone else's.

We tend to ignore hearing loss because it's so much easier than treating it. Once it becomes undeniable, we ignore it because we don't really know what to do about it. Most people don't know where to go for a hearing test. They don't know whether it's an issue for their internist, an ENT, or an audiologist. They're not even sure it's something they should treat or if it's just a natural part of aging. It *is* a natural part of aging, the same way elevated cholesterol and blood pressure are, the same way an arthritic knee is. We treat the high cholesterol and high blood pressure, we do physical therapy for the arthritic knee. Why then do we simply accept hearing loss as inevitable?

Hearing loss is dismissed as a lifestyle problem. Or an attitude problem. We aren't listening closely enough. We aren't paying attention. Spousal hearing loss is a familiar joke: We hear what we want to and ignore the rest.

Even when they finally acknowledge the hearing loss and are told they would benefit from hearing aids, most people don't get them. Only a fraction of those Americans who could benefit from a hearing aid has one. Why don't people use hearing aids? The short answer is stigma, cost, and confusion.

Because it's an invisible disability, hearing loss is easy for others to ignore, too. No one "looks" deaf. When I tell people I have hearing loss, and ask if they can speak more slowly, they don't know how to respond. Do I need a sign language interpreter, they ask? Can I show them the sign for Hello? I don't know sign language. I speak English and have for the past sixty-five years.

They also don't know how to talk to someone with hearing loss. They speak in an exaggerated way, or lean into my ear and talk (where I can't see their lips). I have to tell them how to talk to me. But without a visual clue to remind them of the hearing loss, they often quickly forget I ever mentioned it.

One reason hearing loss is so hard for people to comprehend is that we each experience it differently. There is no "typical" hearing loss. How a person with damaged ears hears depends on dozens of factors, among them the location of the loss (in the hair cells or elsewhere in the ear), the pattern (i.e., how different frequencies are affected), the length of time you've had it, the correction used, his or her particular success with the device, and how well the loss is tolerated emotionally. For some of us, everything is too loud (a condition called recruitment). Others can barely hear sounds. Some of us can't tell a dog's bark from a car backfire, a siren from children shrieking and laughing. Many of us can hear a sentence but not understand a word of it. Some of us are good lip-readers (called speech-reading these days). For others, the ability to speech-read is elusive.

Perhaps the most damaging perception is that hearing isn't that important. When you get old, you lose it. This is an attitude epitomized by the fact that Medicare doesn't cover the cost of hearing aids. Hearing, Medicare seems to be saying, is not essential for healthy aging. And people with hearing loss too often buy into that.

Why Ignorance Is Dangerous

When people learn I have hearing loss, they often say to me, "Oh, me too! I can't hear anyone in a restaurant. But I don't need hearing aids."

They are wrong. The inability to hear speech in noise is not only one of the first signs of hearing loss, but it may be when you most need hearing aids. If you can preserve the hearing in that ear through the use of a hearing aid, you are also preserving the brain's capacity to understand speech. If you ignore that hearing loss, you are depriving your brain of the stimulation it needs to keep on functioning.

We know now about brain plasticity—the brain changes according to the input it gets. If the speech pathways of the brain aren't being used for speech, they're taken over for some other function. The brain doesn't like idle synapses, and it will quickly find another use for them.

You may be putting yourself at risk for cognitive decline. The harder you have to work to hear and understand, the greater the cognitive energy expended. The cognitive reserves that contribute to memory are being borrowed to allow simple hearing. Solid epidemiological studies have shown a statistically significant relation between hearing loss and dementia. We can't exactly prove why this is. We don't know for sure if hearing aids help—because few randomized control trials have been done to test the potential beneficial effect of hearing aids—but some researchers think we will eventually find this to be the case. But why wait until the research comes in? Common sense says that if you're struggling to hear or you're isolating yourself because you're just plain fed up with the effort of being sociable, you're putting yourself at risk. Hearing loss, which is associated with isolation and loneliness, *may* be a risk factor for dementia. Isolation *is* a risk factor for dementia.

Most hearing loss occurs in the inner ear, which is a part of our vestibular system. Because that system regulates balance as well as hearing, untreated hearing loss can have physical consequences, too. Among them is a threefold greater risk for falls, according to several studies, including one funded by the National Institute on Aging. It is well known that among the elderly a fall is often the beginning of the end.

How to Read This Book

This book is about adult-onset hearing loss, which means any hearing loss that occurs after spoken language is learned. It is not about being culturally Deaf, which is defined primarily by the use of sign language—in America, that's American Sign Language (ASL). Those who are Deaf may wear hearing aids or cochlear implants, but their primary language is ASL. Increasingly, "deaf" and "hard of hearing" are linked, and what's good for one group is good for the other.

There is no one simple term for people with hearing loss like mine—people who have serious, adult-onset loss but remain part of the hearing world. We sometimes use the term "deaf," because we are functionally and legally deaf. ("Legally deaf" means we are entitled to protection under the Americans with Disabilities Act.) Canadians use "hard of hearing," more frequently than Americans. "People with hearing loss" is the preferred term in the United States. "Hearing-impaired" is frowned on by activists, as it suggests that the hearing loss defines the whole person, but professionals like audiologists often use it unthinkingly.

In part, this book is for those who are newly encountering hearing loss. Part One, "Facing Facts," is intended for those who may think they have a problem, but can't quite bring themselves to acknowledge it. This section can help them find an audiologist, choose a hearing aid, and learn how to listen more effectively. It also offers information about other kinds of hearing devices that are less expensive than hearing aids. And it suggests ways to make the most of hearing aids.

Part Two, "Love and Work," addresses the issues that arise in daily life for someone with hearing loss, both at home and in the workplace. This section is intended for those who already have hearing aids or a cochlear implant, but who still have difficulties in the hearing world. It discusses family relationships, dating, friendships, and issues that arise at work. Chapter 13, "Mid-Career Hearing Loss, or, My Mistakes," details the issues that arose for me in the workplace over the years, and how I wish I had dealt with them.

Part Three, "Travel and Leisure," suggests ways that people with hearing loss can deal with challenges they face while traveling and in public spaces, like restaurants. It offers suggestions for managing in those situations—as well as suggestions for how we can make those situations more hearing friendly. It also discusses safe driving tips.

Part Four, "When Hearing Aids Aren't Enough," focuses on the issues that come as hearing worsens and hearing aids no longer are sufficient on their own to keep up with an active life. Chapter 19 is about speech-reading, how you can teach yourself, and why it's not always effective. Other chapters address assistive technology to enhance hearing, an area that is booming with innovation.

Part Five, "Changing the Way We Think About Hearing Loss," addresses the underlying ignorance and bias about hearing loss, where it originates, and why it is so persistent. It also reiterates the importance of treating hearing loss, from both a personal and public health perspective.

Overcoming ignorance and stigma means changing our attitudes and our laws. It's not something any one of us can do alone, but as more and more people become open and honest about hearing loss, their needs and their voices will be heard. We're on the cusp of a change in acceptance and treatment of hearing loss. It's exciting to see the old obstacles begin to tumble.

It's also personally gratifying to be part of making that happen. Advocacy is empowering. Rather than being a victim of your disability, you turn it into a tool for change, for change that will benefit you, yes, but also many others.

This book takes the reader through the full experience of hearing loss, from the first inklings that something is wrong, through gradual realization that it's not going away and may in fact be worsening. If hearing does continue to decline, we are eventually faced with the undeniable realization that we have lost something precious, something essential to living fully—and we respond with grief. Thankfully, these days we can usually restore hearing through technology. Not always and not always completely, and sometimes not even well. But by refusing to be stigmatized by it, we begin to accept it.

We find others like ourselves; we begin to realize how many people share our experience. The grief over the loss gives way to acceptance, anger to advocacy. If we're lucky, we learn to laugh at our errors, we make new friends in our new world, and we discover strengths in ourselves.

I hope this book will provide guidelines for people at every stage of the hearing loss journey.

Note: Because a great deal of information is available both in print and online, I've included endnotes to direct those with particular interests to further reading. I've also included a list of resources at the end of the book for those with hearing loss. It's by no means comprehensive, but one thing leads to another on the Web, and these are intended as a starting point.

PART ONE

Facing Facts

I Don't Have Hearing Loss. I Just Can't Hear You.

"Denial is the refusal to acknowledge the existence or severity of unpleasant external realities or internal thoughts and feelings."[1]

Do you have hearing loss? Before you say no, consider these questions:

Are you uncomfortable at meetings because you're not always sure what's said?

Does your spouse complain that the TV is too loud?

Is it difficult to hear your wife when she talks to you as she walks out of the room?

Do you complain about the noise in restaurants?

Is it difficult to hear your watch (nondigital) ticking?

Do you have trouble hearing a whisper?

Do you find that people often say, "Oh, never mind. It's not important"?

It's very easy to dismiss a "yes" answer to any or all of these questions. The world has a problem, not you. You can hear just fine.

In meetings, that guy with the mustache mumbles interminably. The woman from marketing is so shy no one can hear her. Everybody talks at the same time. Everybody talks too fast.

Is the TV too loud? It's those damn commercials.

You can't hear your wife when she walks out of the room? Of course you can't. She's probably just had the last word in a conversation you didn't want to have anyway. Her mind is already on something else and whatever she said was tossed off in parting.

Can't hear in a restaurant? Everybody knows restaurants are too loud.

Can't hear your watch ticking? Do watches tick anymore? Yes, and so do clocks, especially the kind in offices where the minute hand moves forward in a slight jerk.

Whisper? Why is that person hissing in my ear?

That person who says, "Oh, never mind, it's not important"? He probably didn't want you to hear him in the first place and regretted saying whatever it was he said. But if you're getting this fairly regularly, it may be telling you something.

You May Not Notice What You're Missing

Hearing loss can be easy to miss at first. The most common kinds of hearing loss, brought on by exposure to noise or by aging, are gradual. Sometimes people don't even realize they have it until someone (a family member or friend) suggests a hearing test. Even then they may insist they don't have hearing loss, they just can't hear in this restaurant, at this party...whatever. Denial of hearing loss is so powerful that some people fool even themselves.

If I brush my teeth without my hearing aid or cochlear implant (CI), I often forget to turn off the water. I don't hear it. It doesn't seem unusual that I don't hear it. Water running from the tap just seems like something that doesn't make much noise. But then when I put in my hearing aid and turn on the CI, I hear a loud rushing sound from the bathroom. Suddenly, it's Niagara Falls in there.

Think of leaves rustling—you can easily forget it's not only a visual but an aural experience. Or traffic noise. This may be one you'd just as soon not hear, but it's surprising how normal it can seem to see but not hear traffic.

A cat purring. It's a tactile sensation—you feel the vibration. And then you remember that purring is a sound as well. The coffeepot gurgling. With just my hearing aid, I figure the coffeepot is a pretty quiet machine. When I put on my cochlear implant, which picks up lower frequency sounds better than my hearing aid does, I can hear the gurgling well enough to know when the coffee is done. I can also hear the beep at the end of the dishwasher cycle.

If I didn't have hearing aids or an implant, and had only mild to moderate hearing loss, I might not notice that I wasn't hearing these things.

The Age Bias

We think of hearing loss as a natural condition of aging, because the people you most often see with hearing aids are the elderly. Half of the forty-eight million Americans with hearing loss are under fifty-five, but it affects two-thirds of people seventy and over.[2, 3] Those who first experience hearing loss when they are young get older. It is likely to worsen with every decade. As they become less self-conscious about signs of age, they may finally decide to try a hearing aid. Suddenly, the elderly with hearing loss constitute a critical mass.

The $$$$ Deterrent

Hearing aids are expensive. Some people think they are not only expensive but a rip-off. Why can I buy a new smartphone for

$300, they ask, and have to pay ten times that amount for a hearing aid? It's not unusual for an audiologist to sell a hearing aid for $3,000. And because both noise and age-related hearing loss affect both ears, you'll probably need two. The average price for a mid-level pair is $4,400 to $4,500.

Big-box stores like Costco have seen an opportunity in the need for affordable hearing aids. They buy high-end aids in bulk and sell them at a lower cost to the consumer. Costco is now the largest (or one of the largest—the company has been coy on the subject) hearing aid distributor.[4] Online retailers have also jumped into the fray. Thanks to these new sources, the marketplace has changed dramatically. Independent audiologists still play an important role, especially for people with severe hearing loss, but for those with mild to moderate loss the options are much broader than they were even a decade ago.

And what about health insurance? In the past, private and public health insurers have implicitly discouraged the use of hearing aids by not reimbursing for them. Some private insurers are beginning to realize that hearing aids are in fact a cost-effective deterrent of future problems, like dementia. UnitedHealthcare, one of the country's largest insurers, offers affordable hearing aids, beginning at $649, through HiHealth Innovations.[5] AARP offers members hearing aids starting at $795, through HearUSA.[6] Alternatives to traditional hearing aids, PSAPs (covered in Chapter 5), are also becoming an option.

Even with the increase in affordable options, for some, hearing aids are prohibitively expensive. What's the point of diagnosing hearing loss, you think, if I can't afford to treat it? Two good reasons to have your hearing checked have nothing to do with hearing better. The first is that the problem may be something very simple, like wax in your ears, which is easily removed. Or the loss may be a symptom of something serious, the first sign of an autoimmune disorder or cardiovascular disease, or a tumor on your auditory nerve. Something you might be able to treat if you catch it early enough.

Hearing Aids' Bad Rap

The perception that hearing aids don't work is powerful. But they do work! Especially for milder hearing loss. A mild to moderate loss can have a disproportionate effect on your life. You're fine with family and friends. You don't think about your hearing as you go about your daily life. But you can't hear at your place of worship. You can't hear at the movies. You'd like to continue that college course you're auditing but you can't understand the professor well enough. You don't go to lectures anymore.

We remember Grandma's hearing aid whistling and shrieking. And she still said "What?" all the time, or made you talk louder, or just closed her eyes and drifted off. Today's digital hearing aids, however, work very well for many people, even in noise, and they are virtually invisible. And they don't shriek.

Raising the Issue with a Loved One

Being told you have hearing loss is irritating. Most people's instant reaction is a huffy denial.

How do you approach the issue of hearing loss with someone who doesn't want to discuss it? Carefully, cautiously, and specifically.

Instead of pointing out that you've noticed your loved one seems to be missing things, wait until you're sure he's misheard you or someone else and use that as an opener. It's best to do it immediately. If you wait, he has a chance to turn the tables and say it's *you* who's not *remembering* correctly. But it's also best to do it when you're alone. Your loved one may not even let you finish the sentence. "No, I'm not missing anything. I don't have a problem." Or, alternatively, "Of course, I'm missing things, I'm seventy-three. But it doesn't bother me."

Don't be deterred! Rephrase your comment: "It seems *to me* that you're missing some things." Remind your dear family member or friend that hearing loss may be a symptom of something easy to correct, or something important to treat.

It's not going to do much good to insist that the person should be hearing better. The response is a knee-jerk rebuff. More effective is to suggest that, given the possible explanations for the loss, it probably shouldn't be ignored.

Leave it at that, at least until the next time.

For a more devious approach, see the blog post I wrote called "Talking About Hearing Loss to Someone Who Doesn't Want to Listen."[7]

Despite the refusal to acknowledge hearing loss, and no matter how resistant a person may be, she usually has a nagging suspicion that something is wrong. Go back to that list at the beginning of the chapter. If you answered yes to more than one or two of the questions, you may have hearing loss. It could be just be earwax. It might be a symptom of cardiovascular disease or a brain tumor. Don't ignore it. Knowledge is power. Once you know what the problem is, you can choose how to deal with it.

CHAPTER TWO

Get It Tested

It might be hearing loss, or it might not.
The only way to find out is to have it tested.
You don't have to take your wife's word for it.

Where to Start

Many people simply don't know where to go for a hearing test, or what kind of professional they should consult. This is less an indication of their ignorance than it is of the confusing and contradictory hearing-health-care system.

Hearing tests are not routinely given as part of an adult physical. Given the reluctance to acknowledge hearing loss, and a tendency for doctors to underestimate its importance, this means most people never get tested, because it requires taking the active step of finding a place to get one.

Sometimes you don't have to look far. You've probably seen mobile hearing test vans, offering tests at your local mall or a street fair. These are usually free, and offered by qualified professionals. You can often get a hearing test at the audiology department of a nearby university. You can get a test from an audiologist in private practice or from one working with an otolaryngologist. You can go to Costco, Beltone, HearUSA, Miracle-Ear, or any store that has an audiologist on staff. The one place you probably won't get a hearing test is at your primary-care doctor's office.

What you may get at that annual physical is a hearing *screening*,[8] a list of questions (similar to those at the beginning of Chapter 1) that may lead your doctor to suggest you get a full hearing *test*. The doctor should be able to refer you to an ENT with an audiologist on staff, to an independent audiologist, or to an audiologist employed by a store like Costco (though not all stores have audiologists on staff, so check before you go).

Depending on your health insurance, visiting the ENT or independent audiologist may be advantageous financially. Even though the hearing test will be performed by an audiologist with the same license as the audiologist at, say, Costco, your health insurance is more likely to cover it as a medical necessity.

An ENT can also order diagnostic tests to rule out underlying causes of your hearing loss. But if you're fifty or sixty, and your hearing loss is about the same in both ears, you can assume it's probably the result of too much noise combined with some early aging. Going straight to an audiologist is a reasonable choice. Many audiologists do not charge for hearing tests if they lead to the purchase of hearing aids. But as more people are using an audiologist simply for the test and then buy the hearing aid cheaper elsewhere, more audiologists are charging a fee, with prices ranging from $100 to $300.

A Case for Making a Hearing Test Part of the Annual Physical

A small percentage of doctors do screen hearing, and a few offer hearing tests in their offices, but the equipment is expensive and the standard test is time consuming (it takes about 30 minutes), so it's rare. One family physician in Lake Havasu City, Arizona, tried a different model.

Dr. Thomas J. Powers conducted a six-month trial at his family practice. In addition to his wife, the office manager, he has two receptionists and a medical assistant. Over the six-month period, his medical assistant gave a simple hearing screening to everyone over forty who came in for an annual physical. The administration of the test was unremarkable, just another screening tool like taking blood pressure or temperature. Patients also filled out a self-assessment of their hearing. If the patient scored below a certain point on either of these screenings, Dr. Powers asked a few questions to rule out underlying medical causes for the hearing loss, and if the person seemed to be at risk, he recommended a standard "pure-tone" hearing test using a computer program, administered by his wife.

Over the six-month trial, 767 patients were screened. Of these, the screening found that 138 seemed at risk for hearing loss. Within the at-risk group, 107 took the computerized hearing test. Dr. Powers said about 80 percent of those who took the computer test showed signs of age-related loss. (The other 20 percent showed signs of hearing loss that might be indicative of an underlying condition,[9] and they were referred to local ENTs or to the House Clinic in Los Angeles.) As for the 80 percent, Dr. Powers offered them—right then and there, at the appointment—a pair of fairly simple, low-cost hearing aids. He encouraged the patient to try them out during the rest of the physical. The hearing aids were the open fit kind (see Chapter 4, about hearing aids, for a full explanation), which does not require making molds or a precise fitting in the ear canal.

What's surprising is what came next. Forty-four percent of these patients bought their hearing aids. (Compare this to the low figures for hearing aid use overall.) Those who chose not to get hearing aids said either that they couldn't afford them (they were $1,500 for a pair), were not yet ready for hearing aids, or didn't need them. Most who said they didn't need them were older men without their wives present, who had what Dr. Powers called "GOMD"—grumpy old man disease.

In a follow-up questionnaire, 72 percent reported they were wearing their hearing aids eight to sixteen hours a day. This is a notably high rate of use. Most new hearing aid users wear them just a few hours a day, or find them irritating and put them in a drawer.

Several factors may account for the success of Dr. Powers's experiment. First is the routine nature of the hearing screening, which is not announced in advance and is incorporated into the annual physical. The second is the immediate availability of a hearing test and of hearing aids. Both of these approaches help people to overcome the reluctance to get hearing tested or to try hearing aids. The patient doesn't have to make an appointment, make a trip to an audiologist, or wait for delivery of the hearing aids. Every step a person has to take reduces the likelihood of doing anything about a hearing issue.

The lower cost of the hearing aids is also a factor, but a lesser one because you can get hearing aids at that price, or even for less, at a variety of outlets. It's the routine screen and test plus the immediate availability of a product you can try out over the next hour or so of your appointment that makes the difference.

Testing Yourself at Home

You can test your hearing at home, but you won't get precise results. No home hearing test is as accurate as, say, a blood-pressure cuff or a glucometer. But it can be a helpful first step for those who are reluctant to get tested at an audiologist's office.

Many online tests are actually a self-screening, with a list of questions, similar to those in screenings used elsewhere. But for it to work you have to be honest. Put denial on the back burner.

You can find online hearing tests—actual pure-tone tests (the basic hearing test, and a good indication of hearing loss)—by Googling them. Although these are similar to the test an audiologist uses, they're not precise and often not accurate. The beeps (the pure tones) come at regular intervals, and consciously or not you know when to expect the next tone. An audiologist will vary the time between the tones to prevent you from anticipating the next tone.

Most of these self-tests give only the most general responses, such as a recommendation to see an audiologist. They also come with a caveat, like this one, from the hearing aid manufacturer Phonak: "Please be aware that this screening is for informational purposes only and is not intended to replace a professional hearing evaluation. For an accurate measurement of your hearing ability, you should consult with a qualified hearing care professional." If you're reading this on a computer, the link will take you to a page where you fill in your zip code to find an expert near you.

I tried this online test, wearing my hearing devices, and got this result: "It would be recommended that you have your hearing checked properly by a hearing expert."

Some are better than others. Myhearingtest.net offers a simplified pure-tone test. I checked it against my audiologist's audiogram. It was in the same neighborhood: mild to moderate loss (with hearing aid and cochlear implant). If I didn't already know that I had hearing loss, the results of this test would surely have sent me straight to an audiologist.

A promising new telephone-based hearing test, the National Hearing Test, was developed by Communication Disorders Technology, a Bloomington, Indiana, company in partnership with Indiana University and VU University Medical Center in Amsterdam. The participant registers at nationalhearingtest.org and pays \$5 to obtain an access code for use on the toll-free line. But this site, too, carefully notes that it is "not a substitute for a full hearing evaluation by an audiologist." Because hearing loss, especially in only one ear, could be a sign of a condition requiring medical attention, it's important to heed the recommendation to see a specialist. In the case of a sudden hearing loss (you can read more about this in Chapter 6), time is of the essence and medical intervention a must. Sudden hearing loss is a medical emergency.

Considering how many people who suspect they may have hearing loss shove their suspicions to the back of their minds, the easy availability of this test may persuade people to try it out. One of the bigger obstacles to treating hearing loss is the initiative it takes to make that first appointment with an audiologist. But having a home test confirm your suspicions should give you the push you need to reach out.

CHAPTER THREE

Your First Audiologist Appointment

Finding and visiting a good audiologist.

There are several paths that might lead you to an audiologist's office. Perhaps you first visited an ENT and discovered that you need hearing aids. Or maybe you have garden-variety noise- or age-related hearing loss and skipped the ENT altogether. Either way, you're going to need to find a good audiologist.

If your ENT gave you recommendations, you can check the names against a list of professionals certified by the American Speech-Language-Hearing Association (ASHA).[10] The American Academy of Audiology also has a directory where you can choose by geography and specialty. You might also ask others with hearing loss if they like their audiologist. It's surprising how many people don't like their audiologists—or maybe don't even know their names— but stick with them because it's complicated to switch. Try to get a person-centered audiologist, with whom you will be compatible, right from the start. This could be a long-term relationship.

Finding a Good Audiologist

When I asked an expert at a hearing-loss convention about distinguishing the good audiologists from the bad, she replied tartly that there is no such thing as a bad audiologist, just bad patients. Or maybe she softened it a bit by saying just bad relationships.

I beg to differ, as do many of my fellow hearing loss colleagues. There are bad audiologists, just as there are bad doctors and bad teachers and bad psychotherapists. They rush, they make mistakes, they don't listen, they make you wait for two hours, they don't schedule follow-up appointments.

Some don't completely understand or refuse to embrace current technology. They tell you that you don't need a telecoil, they don't know much about hearing assistive technology, they don't want to talk about PSAPs, or they've never heard of induction loops. (These technologies will be discussed in Chapter 18, on assistive listening devices, but for a quick explanation see the Glossary.)

Hearing aid companies own some private practices,[11] and their audiologists will be eager to sell you their company's hearing aid, often without acknowledging the company affiliation. If an audiologist offers only one or two brands of hearing aids, and you don't like what you're offered, try another audiologist.

People often go to doctors or dentists they know through their community or those who have been recommended by other doctors. But most people have never met an audiologist, and most doctors in general or family practices don't know any, either. There's a reason it's hard to find an audiologist: There are not that many to be found. ASHA, which has more audiologists associated with it than any other professional organization, numbers just 14,000 certified audiologists among its members, which also include speech-language pathologists, research scientists, and students.[12] By comparison, there are 2.8 million registered nurses in the United States.

As if diving into the unknown weren't daunting already, the world of audiologists can be very confusing to sort through. An April 2014 survey conducted by the *Hearing Review*[13] demonstrated the wide array of job titles and qualifications in the field of audiology. Among the 179 survey respondents, some called themselves "dispensing audiologists," while others were "hearing-instrument" specialists (who are not audiologists). Their qualifications varied, depending on when they entered practice. Audiologists have either a master's or doctoral degree. The doctoral degree, which became mandatory for new audiologists in 2012, is either a PhD or Doctor of Audiology (AuD). Hearing instrument specialists are not trained as audiologists and in many states need only a high school degree. They must pass a state licensing exam and perform a brief apprenticeship with a licensed hearing aid specialist.[14]

Margaret Wallhagen, a professor of Gerontological Nursing at the University of California, San Francisco,[15] addressed this confusing array of hearing aid specialists at a January 2014 symposium on hearing loss and healthy aging, convened by the Institute of Medicine and the National Research Council. She noted that even within these categories, "Specialists and their corresponding professional associations can also disagree among themselves about the types of service that practitioners should offer, how services should be reimbursed, and the ways services are accessed by patients."

My personal opinion is that while advanced degrees are probably preferable, more important is a patient-centered attitude, a willingness to ask questions and listen to answers, an open mind about alternatives to hearing aids, and a knowledge of assistive devices.

A good audiologist will assess your hearing needs, and your fears and frustrations. Good audiologists will have incorporated good listening behaviors into their general approach. For instance, after determining that you do in fact have hearing loss but before barraging you with information, the audiologist should give you an opportunity to talk about your worries and expectations about treating your hearing loss. Open-ended questions invite you to be more specific and help avert dissatisfaction later on. "Before we talk about the details of your hearing test, do you have any questions for me?" the audiologist might ask. "Have you talked to others about hearing loss and hearing aids?" She might ask if you've looked into telephone amplifiers or if you use captions when you watch TV.

The audiologist may also try to determine at this point how motivated the patient is. Has a wife dragged in her husband, who insists that he's fine? Sometimes patients come in voluntarily to talk about their hearing loss but are not psychologically ready for hearing aids. Ambivalence is common, and the audiologist has to recognize how far to push a patient. Prematurely prescribing hearing aids will probably not have optimal results: They're likely to end up at the bottom of that drawer. An audiologist should be assessing your readiness or motivation, as these are predictors of success.

A good audiologist should give you only the amount of information you can absorb. A number of studies in all kinds of health-care settings have shown that patients have poor retention of information given them in an appointment. Patients are under some emotional stress—they have just had their hearing loss confirmed and have been told that they should get hearing aids. Not the best circumstances for retaining a lot of new and technical information. It always helps to have another person with you, but it also helps if the audiologist limits the amount of information in the first visit, and invites you back for a second consultation after you've had a chance to process the initial information. Always ask for written material to review later.

The relationship with your audiologist does not end with buying and fitting your hearing aids. He will need to see you over the first few months, recalibrating the settings as your brain becomes accustomed to hearing again. In the first months with a new device, the audiologist may set the hearing aid below the anticipated final level of amplification to allow your ear and brain to gradually adapt. At a later visit, he may set them above the target level: I learned to walk out of the audiologist's office with my hearing aids programmed just a little louder than was comfortable because I knew by the next day (and in the outside world) they would sound right.

A good audiologist should also encourage you to give the hearing aids a real try, to wear them as much as possible when you're awake. Some people may need to start with just a few hours and gradually increase the time. Others may want to plunge in and wear them all day. If you don't make this concerted effort—if you just put them on when you go to the movies—you're not getting anything close to the benefits you could be. But it takes time to recognize these benefits. If you rarely wear your hearing aids, you'll probably never get to the point of appreciating them.

It's also important for an audiologist to gauge your emotional response to your newly diagnosed hearing loss. The audiologist should know about support groups like the Hearing Loss Association of America (HLAA) and the Association of Late-Deafened Adults (ALDA), and be able to refer you to local chapters.

In the public-health sector, you may get one shot at an audiologist. The U.S. Department of Veterans Affairs (VA) provides free hearing aids and hearing accessories to servicemen and servicewomen. In some VA facilities, audiologists don't have the time to provide much in the way of counseling or rehabilitation. It may be a fitting, and then good-bye. Come back in six months and we'll see how you're doing. At that point, they may adjust the programming or even recommend aural rehabilitation (see Chapter 7). Others, for instance the Manhattan and Brooklyn VAs, schedule more frequent follow-ups, and the patient can also ask for an appointment.

Finally, don't forget to make sure the office is not too hard to get to. If you get hearing aids, you should be spending a lot of time with your audiologist over the first few months.

Before You Go

Most audiologists have a busy schedule, and you'll probably have to wait for a first appointment. If you're on the fence about whether you're ready for hearing aids, just schedule it. And don't forget to cancel if you change your mind. The initial appointment will probably take an hour or more, because there's a lot of ground to cover. Follow-ups will be easier to schedule and will be shorter.

Whether your appointment is with an audiologist in private practice, at a doctor's office or hospital, with a hearing aid vendor, or at a big-box store like Costco, be prepared.

You'll be providing and receiving a lot of information, so if possible take someone along with you to help. Make a list of all your medications and dosages, as well as any hearing and non-hearing health issues you have now, or have had in the past. Make a list of questions you want to ask the audiologist. Write down where you have the most problems hearing and understanding, and what you hope to gain from hearing aids.

The first visit will probably start with an interview (the lists will expedite things). The audiologist will ask about your general health history, your work history, your exposure to noise, the kinds of medications you take or have taken. She will also of course ask about your hearing. How long ago did you notice you weren't hearing as well as you used to? In what kinds of situations do you find it most difficult to hear? What are the hearing challenges you face on a daily basis? For instance, if you work, is acute hearing an essential part of the job? Do you have young children or elderly or sick relatives at home whom you need to be able to hear if they call out at night?

If you think in advance about these questions, you may realize you've overlooked information that initially seemed irrelevant to your hearing loss. Medical history may either help explain the loss or give the audiologist a sense of what kind of hearing assistance would work best for you.

We don't all have the same hearing needs. A working professional probably requires more precise hearing than a factory worker. Teachers or psychotherapists rely on sharp hearing in their work. Hospital employees may frequently need to understand patients or physicians wearing surgical masks, which prevents supplementing hearing by reading lips. A retiree may care most about being able to talk on the telephone to her children or watch TV. A birdwatcher may be frustrated by his inability to hear birdcalls, or to locate them if he can hear them. We each have specific requirements and priorities.

Tests and Procedures

After the initial conversation, an audiologist will do a brief physical exam. He will take a look at your ear with an otoscope to make sure nothing visible is affecting your hearing. If wax is impacting the ear, he may remove it (never try this yourself—you'll only shove it in deeper). Some audiologists will refer you to a doctor for wax removal.

No matter what kind of screening or testing you've had previously, the audiologist will want to do her own testing.

He'll escort you into a soundproof booth with a heavy door and a thick window to an adjoining room. My audiologist uses the same rooms for testing children and adults, and I often sit in a child-size chair at a child-size table, with a box of toys nearby. (The toys are tools for measuring hearing in young children. The child is told to add a block whenever he hears a sound.) The booth itself is a little like a large walk-in refrigerator, though not as cold. If you have a tendency to claustrophobia, you may want to ask the audiologist if the door can be left open. This decreases the soundproofing but if there isn't too much ambient noise in the hallway, it should be fine.

Several different tests may be done at the appointment. How many depends on your hearing. If you test normal on the first one, that may be it, especially if the audiologist has also removed earwax that may have contributed to your sense of hearing loss.

The Pure-Tone Air- and Bone-Conduction Tests

Often, the first test audiologists will do is what's called a pure-tone test, one ear at a time.[16] It measures how loud you need a sound to be before you can hear at a specific frequency (pitch). This is called your hearing threshold (the pure-tone is also called a threshold test). Loudness (more accurately, perception of intensity) is expressed in decibels; a person with normal hearing can hear at between 10 and 25 decibels. Frequency is expressed in hertz; the lowest frequency humans can hear is 250 Hz and the highest is 20,000. Most hearing loss varies across the frequencies. For instance, you might hear when the sound is just 20 decibels in the lower frequencies but you need the level raised to 50 decibels to hear in the mid frequencies.

Most speech sounds are found between 500 and 4,000 hertz.

The first part of the pure-tone procedure is an air-conduction test. You'll put on a set of headphones or earphones and face the audiologist, visible through the window. She will play a series of tones at different frequencies, and at different decibel levels, watching to see how you respond. The test usually begins at 1,000 hertz, a mid frequency, but it can be lower, depending on the audiologist's preference. When you hear a tone, you signal to the audiologist by raising a finger, by saying "yes," or by pressing a hand-held device. (For toddlers, it's stacking a block.) The booth should be set up so that you cannot see what the audiologist is doing, because that would be a visual tip-off that could skew the results.

The test is usually administered manually, which means the audiologist is activating the tones. They come at irregular intervals, which is one reason these tests are more accurate than online tests. Online versions play the tones at regular intervals, and it's easy to guess—even subconsciously—when to press the button.

The tones usually begin at about a 30-decibel level for someone who thinks he may have hearing loss. The first tone should be higher than what the patient could be expected to hear, given his hearing history. If you can hear the tone at 25 decibels, your hearing is close to normal—a very mild loss. The object is to find the softest level at which you can hear the sounds, so don't worry if the sounds are very soft; the audiologist is doing this on purpose.

You're going to want to pay full attention—no drinking, chewing gum, or squirming. Sometimes you won't be sure if you've heard a tone or not, which can result in a false positive if you press the signal when there's no sound. A false negative comes when the subject hears the tone but fails to press the signal at the expected levels. Each frequency is tested several times to compensate for false positives or negatives.

Next comes the bone-conduction test, which determines whether your hearing problem is in the inner ear or is caused by blockage or damage in the outer or middle ear. An inner ear problem is called sensorineural hearing loss. A blockage or malfunction in the middle or outer ear is called conductive hearing loss. (A mixed hearing loss occurs when you have a combination of the two.) For the bone-conduction test, the audiologist will come into the soundproof booth and fit you with a different headset. It can feel awkward or uncomfortable, especially where the measuring instrument presses on the bone behind the ear. Once the audiologist places the bone vibrator at the correct spot, you shouldn't move for the rest of the test.

If the bone-conduction test result is normal and shows a better result than the air-conduction test, that suggests that your problem is in the middle or outer ear: The sound is not getting through to cochlea.

Other tests may or may not be done. One that usually is performed is tympanometry, which measures how well the middle ear is performing its job.

Speech Perception Tests

Even if your hearing test is normal, the audiologist will move on to testing your speech perception. (The test is called the "speech reception threshold," abbreviated SRT.) He reads a list of familiar two-syllable words—like ice cream, playground, and airplane—hiding his mouth so you can't read his lips. I've had this test so many times I can probably recite all the words from memory. It determines the lowest level at which the patient can correctly identify 50 percent of common two-syllable words. The levels should be pretty close to the levels on the pure-tone test.

The second level of testing is word recognition, which can be a challenge. Using a recording, the audiologist first determines the correct and comfortable volume for presenting the words. A recorded voice takes it from there. Here's what this test is like for me.

Ready? the recording says. I look blankly at the audiologist behind the soundproof glass. She waves at me.

Ready? Say the word Sheep, the calm recorded voice says.

Cheap, I say.

Ready? Say the word Mess.

Mesh?

Ready? Say the word Witch.

Wish? Rich?

The recording is relentless, never pausing while you think of the right answer. Sometimes it feels like an aural Rorschach test. I find myself blurting out words I know can't be correct, that no one would ever use on a test.

Ready? Say the word Juice.

Jews? No, no, that can't be right.[17]

Ready? Say the word Sit.

Shit. No, no, no!

Sometimes I can't even get them out of my mouth they're so inappropriate.

This test is a measure of how well you understand speech when the sound level is set appropriately for your hearing loss. "Appropriately" means that the sounds are presented a level above your "quiet conversation" level. If your hearing is normal, that would be at about 45dB. It helps the audiologist decide on the next steps to take in managing your hearing.

The ability to understand speech is not always predictable from the pure-tone test, and it is not related to how the hearing loss is affecting your daily function. Ask the audiologist to test how well you understand speech in noise (like in a restaurant), as this is probably why you came in for a hearing test in the first place.

How to Read the Audiogram

The results of all these tests are recorded on a single sheet of paper: the audiogram. After the tests, the audiologist will show you the audiogram and discuss what it means. It's taken me years to figure out how to read one, especially because they tend to vary. The following page shows one of my audiograms, taken in 2008, just before I received my cochlear implant.

The largest box, in the upper left corner, shows my pure-tone test results. Frequencies are listed horizontally, left to right, at the top, with the lowest frequency at the left. Decibel levels are listed vertically, with the lowest decibel level at the top. An x symbolizes the hearing in your left ear and a circle represents the hearing in your right ear. As you can see in my chart, the hearing in my pre-implant left ear is significantly worse than my right.

An audiogram of someone with normal hearing will show a more or less flat line across the frequencies at between 10 and 20 decibels. The audiogram of someone with hearing loss will show responses below normal hearing, sometimes sloping or jagged, as mine does here. In noise- or age-related loss, for instance, you can usually hear well in the low frequencies, up to about 1,000 hertz—that is, 50 percent of the

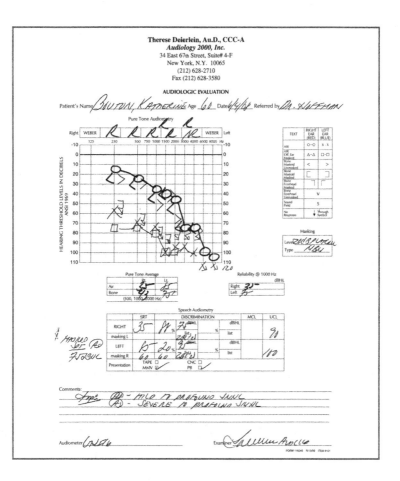

Therese Deierlein, Au.D., CCC-A
Audiology 2000, Inc.
34 East 67th Street, Suite# 4-F
New York, N.Y. 10065
(212) 628-2710
Fax (212) 628-3580

AUDIOLOGIC EVALUATION

Patient's Name *BOUTON, KATHERINE* Age *60* Date *4/4/08* Referred by *Dr. Hoffman*

time you were able to hear the tone at between 10 and 20 decibels. But at 2,000 hertz, your ability to hear requires louder tones, so the line begins to slope steadily down toward the bottom of the chart. It typically hovers in the middle frequencies (2,000–4,000 hertz) at 30 to 50 decibels, and then drops again in the high frequencies (4,000–8,000 hertz) to a point where you need the tones to reach 60 or 70 decibels to hear them. (Audiologists don't generally test above 8,000 hertz.) The audiologist may take an average of your hearing in the mid frequencies (500, 1,000, and 2,000 Hz) and use that to describe the severity of hearing loss.

As you can see in my chart, I needed the decibel level cranked a bit higher throughout, but my audiogram generally follows this sloping pattern, dropping dramatically after the 1,000 Hz and 4,000 Hz benchmarks.

Someone who needs the decibel level turned up to 70 dB before he can hear a sound has a severe hearing loss, but he does not have a 70 percent loss. This is a misconception that is often repeated, probably because it's easier to grasp than the truth. Neil Bauman,[18] author and the director of the Center for Hearing Loss Help, who also publishes the popular HearingLossHelp.com website, describes it this way: "I have a 70 dB loss. This is not equal to a 70 percent loss by any means. In actual fact, it means that the softest sound I can hear needs to be 10,000,000 times louder than the softest sound a person with normal hearing can hear."

This may sound implausible, but decibels increase exponentially. An increase of 10 means that a sound is 10 times more intense, or powerful. To your ears, it sounds twice as loud. The sound of an ambulance siren at 120 decibels is about 1 trillion times more intense than the weakest sound our ears can hear. Bauman goes on: "Quite a difference, isn't it? Now you can see why we must never use percentages when talking about our hearing losses. They just do not equate. They are absolutely meaningless!"[19] (A percentage is used to quantify speech perception: For instance, I may understand 75 percent of words at a particular decibel level.)

The rest of the audiogram typically shows the results of the tympanogram, which measures the health of the eardrum, and the speech tests. On my audiogram, you can see the results of my speech threshold test in the lower box, where it says "SRT" (Speech Recognition Threshold) and the results of my word recognition test under "Discrimination." At the bottom, the audiologist usually records his general impressions.

In 1988, when I was first hired at *The New York Times*, I was given a routine physical, which included a not-so-routine hearing test. The audiogram showed that I had normal hearing in the right ear but the left was a jagged slope with the loss ranging from mild to profound. The audiologist's comment was: "Neurological ASAP." An uneven loss like mine can be a red flag for an auditory nerve tumor, and I was immediately sent to an ENT, who sent me for an MRI.

I wasn't surprised or concerned, because I'd known about the hearing loss for a decade. But just to be safe I had the "neurological." The MRI was normal.

When I discovered my initial loss in 1978, it was diagnosed as Sudden Hearing Loss: a loss of 30 decibels over three consecutive frequencies in less than seventy-two hours. Most Sudden Hearing Loss is only in a single ear, and it's almost always sensorineural. Mine matched that description.

But time and progressive loss ruled out this and many other diagnoses. My hearing loss was idiopathic, cause unknown. By 2002, the right ear had joined the left in a steady decline, down to moderate to profound loss. It was then that I first got hearing aids, one in each ear. Five years later, the hearing in my left ear had dropped to profound levels across all the frequencies, and I stopped wearing that hearing aid because it wasn't doing any good.

My ENT recently casually referred to my hearing loss as being caused by Ménière's—a disease of the vestibular system in the inner ear that can cause hearing loss (usually fluctuating loss), vertigo, fullness in the ear, and tinnitus. I have only some of the symptoms— my hearing loss does fluctuate, though it mostly just gets worse, and I have had severe and persistent vertigo. It was oddly comforting to put a name to my condition, but it's meaningless. Because we don't know what caused the Ménière's (if that's what it is), I'm still left with an idiopathic diagnosis—cause unknown.

You might notice that it took me twenty-five years from the time my hearing loss was first diagnosed to the time I got hearing aids. What took me so long? Denial, ignorance, bias. Stupidity, essentially.

CHAPTER FOUR

Hearing Aids: So Many Choices

The possible combinations of style, brand, and features number in the hundreds.

Finding the Hearing Aid That's Right for You

art of what an audiologist does is assess how precisely you need to hear on a daily basis, including how often you plan to wear your hearing aids and for what purposes. If you work in a busy office with frequent staff meetings, or if you interact with clients, patients, or students, or do a lot of work on the telephone, you probably need the best even if your hearing loss is fairly mild. That generally means the most features, which may or may not translate into the most expensive hearing aids.

There are caveats to this, however. As David Kirkwood, who writes about hearing health care on the website Hearing Health &

Technology Matters,[20] explained to me, just saying "most expensive" ignores a lot of factors. "Depending on where you go for your hearing aids, you can pay much more or much less for essentially the same hearing aids. The extra cost may pay for more time and service from the professional involved—or it may just add to his/her profit margin." For example, Costco sells "high-end" hearing aids that would be the most expensive if you went to an audiologist in private practice. Costco has the advantage of buying in bulk, and of not incurring the many costs associated with running a private audiology practice.

But what if you're a carpenter, a house painter, a novelist, or an artist? What if you telecommute? If your job entails working alone most of the time and you just want to hear better at social gatherings, you can probably get away with a hearing aid that has fewer features. Again, the price varies with different vendors.

If you are elderly, and have trouble manipulating small devices, you may want a hearing aid with a remote control rather than a small volume dial on the aid itself, or maybe a hearing aid with automatic volume and programming adjustments. You'll need a large enough battery and battery door to hold the battery securely between your fingers as you insert it. (Better yet, ask your audiologist for the little magnet that you can use to insert and remove the battery. This can save you a lot of lost batteries and unnecessary frustration.) Even with good fine-motor coordination, I sometimes drop my battery—#13, the size of a baby's fingernail—which then rolls under an immovable piece of furniture or down the sink drain. The battery space is designed to be as small as possible, because people want small hearing aids. In fact all hearing aids these days are small, and most are close to invisible, so size should not be an issue.

The Four Main Hearing Aid Styles

Hearing aid styles are designated with a babel of terms and an alphabet soup of abbreviations.[21] Different sources sometimes use different terms for the same style. The terms are often vague and sometimes even misleading. Most sources narrow the style range to four—BTE, ITE, ITC, and CIC—and refer to them by initials, not by name. I'll spell each out below:

BTE, Behind the Ear

Right off, the description is confusing. *Behind the Ear* is a misnomer because this style of hearing aid often has two components: a small banana-shaped processor behind the ear connected by a thin plastic tube or wire to a receiver *in the ear*. Traditional BTEs have the receiver in the case behind the ear and no in-the-ear component, but this is rare now.

The BTE is used for varying degrees of hearing loss, ranging from mild to severe or profound. Depending on the severity and nature of your hearing loss, the in-the-ear component may be a small "dome," in which case the style is called an open-fit hearing aid. Or it may be a snug-fitting custom-made unit.

Open-fit hearing aids are very popular and almost invisible. They don't cause any feeling of fullness in the ear because the dome allows sound waves to pass through the ear canal. Open-fit wearers also find that their own voice sounds more natural. You can usually get these kinds of open-fit BTEs very quickly, because they don't require custom ear molds. They can be just as expensive as the custom-mold variety, however, and have the same internal circuitry.

For more severe loss, the custom-mold BTE will work better. This is a subcategory of BTE known as RIC (receiver in the canal) or RITE (receiver in the ear). This is the style of hearing aid I have. The in-the-ear part is still a small component, and mostly invisible, but it is custom made to fit snugly into your ear canal, which is important for people with severe hearing loss. It goes easily into the ear and is removed by tugging gently on a small plastic antenna-like knob.

With custom-made earpieces, perfect fit is essential. The audiologist injects a pink or green silicone substance into the ear canal and waits five minutes for it to harden. Then he tugs the silicone out and what's in his hand is a mold of your ear. The mold plus your audiogram are sent to the manufacturer. A week or two later you go back to the audiologist to get your new hearing aid.

The resulting ear mold may be that yucky beige color or clear or even glittery, and the behind-the-ear component is typically brushed silver, though you may have a choice of colors. It's pretty much a worry-free device, but you have to be careful not to get it wet. It's so low-maintenance that I often forget it's there when I take a shower or go swimming. Luckily, no disasters so far. But it takes only one complete immersion to destroy the hearing aid. (Many audiologists recommend taking out insurance against damage or loss. Your homeowner's insurance may cover the hearing aids.)

The in-the-ear piece tends to slip a bit if my ear is sweaty, and the plastic tubing sometimes likes to curl the wrong way, meaning the behind-the-ear component ends up dangling next to my ear. But I can persuade it to go back where it belongs. The space behind my ear is crowded, because I also wear glasses. It's even more crowded on the ear with the cochlear implant, with its much larger earpiece. Despite the good fit, my hearing aid whistles if someone greets me with a cheek kiss on the hearing aid side or if I put my head down (for a quick nap, say) on that side.

My BTE/RIC, with a behind-the-ear component and a custom-fitted earpiece in the canal, cost $3,000. The *Hearing Review* reported that this subset of BTEs makes up 58 percent of the hearing aid market and is the most expensive kind of hearing aid, with prices ranging from $1,694 to $2,993.[22] The range in price reflects the sellers—sellers rather than manufacturers set prices—and the number of features on the aid.

A similar style but with a larger custom-fit mold is known as a RITA or "receiver in the aid." Prices for these more traditional hearing aids start at $1,580 and can go as high as $2,769, according to *Hearing Review*. The larger ear mold is easy to clean and, because the hearing aid tends to be very powerful, it needs room for larger batteries with a long life. If possible, the earpiece should be vented to prevent the ear from feeling plugged up (it's sometimes not possible if the user requires an especially powerful aid). While more visible than the kind I have, RITA hearing aids are very effective for kids or adults with severe to profound hearing loss.

Traditional BTEs, without the in-the-ear component, make up 19 percent of the market and range in cost from $1,580 to $2,769, according to the 2014 *Hearing Review* survey.[23]

ITE, In the Ear

ITEs fit into the ear canal, filling all or part of the pinna (the outer ear), and are custom made for a perfect fit. Often called "full shell," they are similar to the RITA in that all components, including the receiver, are in the earmold of the hearing aid. In this style, however, there is no behind-the-ear component. They are usually large enough to allow for features like a telecoil, directional microphones, memory programs, and volume control (for more details on these, see the section "Key Features"). *Hearing Review* gives the price range as $1,600 to $2,757 per hearing aid. They may not work as well as the BTE for someone with very severe loss, but they are appropriate for mild to moderate loss, and sometimes for severe loss depending on the strength of the receiver.

The first hearing aids I had were this in-the-ear style, each one was a small, hard acrylic device. The left was blue and the right was red. They were translucent and looked a little like jewels. They cost as much as jewels, too—$6,000 for the pair, back in 2002. (Sometimes the price is slightly lower if you buy a pair, for any of the styles.) The popularity of this style has dropped in favor of open-fit BTEs with their slim casings.

The ITE did not work very well for the more severe loss in my left ear. (To be fair, today's better technology might have made the aid more useful for me.) I heard basically nothing with it, though because I did have fair low frequency hearing, it gave me a sense of more balanced hearing and was helpful in figuring out which direction a noise was coming from. The aid in the right ear gave me almost normal hearing for six or eight years until my hearing dropped again. After that, it wasn't powerful enough.

ITC, In the Canal

ITC is a small version of the In-the-Ear. It fits deep in the ear canal and consists of a custom-made acrylic shell holding all the electronics. This model is good for people with mild to moderately severe hearing loss. Because the microphone is at the opening of the ear canal, it takes advantage of the normal acoustics of the outer ear. ITCs, which make up 7 percent of the market, range from $1,716 to $2,861 each.

CIC, Completely in the Canal

CICs fit even more deeply in the ear canal than the ITC and for that reason are invisible. The smallest hearing aids you can get, CICs are expensive (the range: $1,695 to $2,958) because the circuitry is so small. They fit close to the eardrum, and because of that proximity need less power to transmit the signal. This style usually doesn't have enough space for a telecoil and is also too small to include a directional microphone. But wind noise can be less of a problem, and some people report that sound is more natural and it provides for slightly better directional hearing than the ITE or ITC. They also have a smaller battery, which means a shorter life and more frequent battery changing. According to AARP's "Consumer Guide to Hearing Aids,"[24] CICs also need more frequent maintenance and cleaning, and thus more visits to the audiologist.

People who don't want to deal with an external hearing aid have an option of several implanted devices. The extended-wear Lyric, now owned by Sonova, is placed entirely inside the ear canal and is worn twenty-four hours a day, seven days a week, by people with mild to moderately severe hearing loss. You do not change the battery or remove the aid from the ear. When the battery is depleted—after two to four months—the audiologist will remove the hearing aid and replace the battery. Even though the aid is water resistant, it is not waterproof. For swimming, you'll need a custom-made earplug to protect the device. Because the Lyric hearing aid has to be replaced, the consumer buys a "subscription," which comes to about $3,000 a year per pair.[25]

The Esteem hearing implant, made by Envoy Medical, is inserted surgically into the middle ear. It's very expensive ($30,000 for the implant itself as well as tests and surgery) and it's fairly new to the market, having received FDA approval in 2010. Although the manufacturer calls it an "implant," the FDA calls it a hearing aid, and it is not covered by Medicare or most other insurance. Some say it improves hearing for those with moderate to severe hearing loss better than a conventional aid does.

One advantage that struck me as possibly worth the inconvenience and cost with implantable aids is that you wear them twenty-four hours a day, which means that you can hear at night when you are in bed. The Esteem has a battery life of four-and-a-half to nine years, after which the battery is replaced in a minor surgical procedure.[26]

You don't need to go as far as having a hearing aid implanted or paying $30,000 to achieve invisibility. Almost all hearing aids are nearly invisible these days, especially the in-the-ear types. Even those with a behind-the-ear component are not noticeable unless you're bald or wear your hair in a style that exposes the back of the ears.

Why Cost Varies

You may wonder why each of these hearing aids comes in a wide range of prices. This is partly because each brand offers different features but also because manufacturers don't set the prices. That decision is left up to the retailer. That's one reason why you may see the very same hearing aid for sale online for $1,365 that your audiologist is selling for $1,600.

There's another reason you might see a different price at the specialist's office. Your audiologist is selling a package that also includes a range of services. The basic cost, which may or may not be the same price you see online, is the device itself plus the cost of fitting and dispensing the hearing aid. A "bundled" price may include follow-up visits, cleaning costs, counseling, and group or individual auditory rehabilitation.

Bundling is a big issue among audiologists right now, as they see business slipping away to the big-box stores and online retailers. A recent article on the website of the American Speech-Language-Hearing Association[27] discussed many challenges audiologists face if they choose to unbundle and charge for each service separately. My hearing aids have always come as part of a bundled package, and I've certainly taken advantage of follow-up visits, cleaning, counseling, and so on. I can't imagine my audiologist has ever made much money on me.

Increasingly, audiologists are starting to see consumers who have bought hearing aids online or at big-box stores and need follow-up services. The fee scale varies, but it is usually several hundred dollars covering a certain number of visits or period of time, with an extra charge for any accessories.

What Are Audiologists Making on That $3,000 Hearing Aid?

Lots of people—especially vociferous and usually anonymous Web commentators—think audiologists are making a killing. This is not the case. A *Hearing Review* survey found that the average independent hearing aid dispenser sold twenty-three hearing aids a month. (The survey excluded any retailer selling more than one hundred units a month, which ruled out the six major retailers, including the big-box stores.) The net profit margin for the dispensers surveyed ranged from 20 percent to 33 percent, with the larger businesses making the larger profits.

A good audiologist won't pressure you into purchasing the most expensive hearing aid but will help you navigate the vast array of choices and find which one is right for you. A good audiologist will also tell you how long the trial period is, and that you should feel free to bring back the hearing aid and try another one if the first is not right for you.

Key Features

The performance of hearing aids has improved immensely in the past two decades. Despite their decreasing size, most have room for a number of features that enhance the listening experience.

Batteries. Almost all hearing aids use small disposable batteries. When I say small, I mean tiny, half the size of your fingernail. If you have stiff, rheumatic fingers or poor vision or any kind of palsy, you want a hearing aid with the largest batteries. This is something the audiologist should take into consideration right from the start. Your hearing aid will come with enough batteries for a few weeks. Batteries can be bought at drugstores, electronics stores, through AARP, online at Amazon.com, and at some big-box stores. They're expensive so keep your eye out for deals. There are also differences in quality across manufacturers, so ask your audiologist which is the best brand to purchase. Also ask if the audiologist provides promotions or special programs for patients.

Batteries last anywhere from a few days to two weeks, depending on the quality, size, and type of battery, the hearing aid's circuitry, and environmental conditions. Whenever you take the hearing aid out, you should open the battery door. This not only saves battery life but, more important, keeps the battery from emitting a high-pitched squeal that you may not hear but your family and dog certainly will. You'll also save battery life if you keep them in the original packaging with the paper tab attached until you're ready to use them. Once the tab is removed the battery begins to drain.

Batteries come in various sizes, to fit specific hearing aids. The sizes don't seem to have any logical terminology: They come in 675, 312, 13, 10, and 5. Many batteries are color-coded. Size 10 is yellow, 312 is brown, 13 is orange, 5 is red, and 675 is blue. My BTE uses 13s. My old BTE used 312s. The higher numbers don't necessarily correspond to a larger size or longer life. It's random. That being said, the 675 is the largest, having the longest life, and is used for the most powerful hearing aids. The smaller the hearing aid, the smaller the battery, and the more costly.

Telecoil. Also called a T-coil, and originally known as a Telephone Coil, the telecoil is an essential component for anyone with hearing loss, even the mildest kind, although some audiologists still do not seem to realize this. Seventy percent of hearing aids now have telecoils, according to a 2014 survey published in the *Hearing Review*.[28]

You may not appreciate it immediately but as you become more familiar with the hearing aid, you'll find that the T-coil has many uses, including the original use of making telephone calls clearer. (For a full description of the telecoil and its uses, see Chapter 18.)

If your audiologist doesn't mention a telecoil, ask about it. But if invisibility is your primary concern—and you use, say, completely-in-the-canal (CIC) aids—you might not want a telecoil, because the kind of assistive devices that work with a telecoil are generally visible. You probably can't get a telecoil anyway, because of the hearing aid's small size.

There is one invisible assistive technology that works with telecoils: the induction loop. I'll talk about looping more in Chapter 20, but here's a quick primer: Looping is a wireless technology that can bring a speaker's voice straight into your ear simply by flipping the telecoil switch on your hearing aid. Even people without hearing problems report that they hear better at lectures, religious services, or the theater using a loop system. Hearing people wear a headset plugged into a loop receiver. People with hearing loss need nothing more than the hearing aids they're already wearing.

Once you get hearing aids with a telecoil, make sure your audiologist activates it and tells you how to use it. It's surprising how many audiologists skip this step.

Directional microphones. Most hearing aids come with directional microphones, which you can activate to improve speech understanding in a noisy situation. Many are automatic. They work by amplifying sound in front of the wearer, minimizing sounds from behind.

Feedback suppression. This feature is supposed to prevent squeals or whistles when the hearing aid gets too close to the phone or when the device doesn't fit well in the ear. The more amplification you need the harder it is to eliminate feedback altogether, but in general hearing aids have come a long way since Grandpa's day when it comes to minimizing feedback. For most people, that is. I have such a strong hearing aid that I cannot cup my hand around my ear, not even touching it, without a squeal. This is a problem with cheek kissing.

Data logging. This feature allows the audiologist to monitor the ways you are using the hearing aid (for instance, whether you use the speech-in-noise program) and amount of time you are wearing it, to make sure you're wearing it enough hours in the day to make a positive difference in your life.

Low-battery alert. My hearing aid beeps when the battery is about to go dead. It sometimes makes me jump, but no one else can hear it. After half an hour, if I've ignored it, it beeps again. I am irrationally irritated by the beep, which always seems to come at an inopportune moment, but it's valuable. My cochlear implant has a similar feature, with a much less annoying tone. It took me a few weeks to recognize the brief high-pitched tone as the low-battery alert.

Manual volume control means that you can turn the volume up or down by a small dial on the hearing aid or by a remote. I have an automatic volume control on my hearing aid but often find that background noise outside is too loud. Recently, the audiologist gave me a remote to try out. It controls the volume and also the programs. I bought it, for $275. Mostly, my hearing aid is adequate in the default setting, but I do turn the volume up in certain situations, like lectures. Some new hearing aids have control apps that allow you to use your smartphone to control your hearing aid. One advantage to this is that you see the volume on the smartphone, as well as hear it.

Many people, especially those with mild to moderate loss, prefer the automatic volume control. It's also better for older people with cognitive difficulties.

Wax guard. Earwax is a major cause of problems with hearing aids, and most hearing aids come with a filter or guard. This is a tiny white plastic trap that fits into the ear end of your hearing aid and helps protect the innards of the device from earwax. It comes attached to a matchstick-shaped piece of plastic, with one end for detaching the new guard, the other end for disposing of the old one. The guard is tiny and easy to drop, at which point it disappears—usually not into the wastebasket, which is what I'm aiming for. The audiologist will give you handfuls. They last forever. Once I thought I'd lost several of the little white pellets in my ear. The audiologist took a look and assured me they were not rattling around inside.

Bluetooth. Many hearing aids can be paired with Bluetooth devices to bring the sound directly into the aid. This usually requires a streamer, which is an extra device that I'll discuss in Chapter 18, about hearing assistive technologies. (Bluetooth also requires a telecoil.) Several hearing aid manufacturers have introduced hearing aids that link directly to Bluetooth-equipped devices, like a smartphone.

Bluetooth is a rapidly developing technology. Cellular communications and Bluetooth were developed to match but not exceed the fidelity of a land line. But as more and more voice traffic is cell-to-cell, providers are changing the technology and more than doubling the fidelity. This clearer sound is a benefit to the hard of hearing. If possible, be sure any device you buy with Bluetooth is labeled Bluetooth 4.0 or HD.

The "Big Six" Brands

For the past decade or so, after a flurry of consolidations in the early 2000s, the dominant hearing aid manufacturers have been known as "the big six."[29] Here's a quick rundown:

GN ReSound, owned by the Danish company GN Store Nord AS, sells a variety of hearing aids in more than eighty countries. The same hearing aid might go by different names, depending on where you are. The ReSound LiNX is iPhone-compatible and can wirelessly stream music from phone to hearing aid.

ReSound owns Beltone, one of the largest retail chains in the United States, which sells ReSound hearing aids under the Beltone brand name. ReSound also sells a brand known as Interton.

Siemens AG, a publicly held German multinational engineering and electronics conglomerate, recently sold its hearing aid division, Audiology Solutions, to EQT VI, a Swedish investment company. According to Siemens AG, the "Siemens product brand" for hearing aids will continue to be available, as the company put it, "over the medium term."

Sonova is a Swiss-based company that owns Phonak, a major manufacturer of hearing aids and hearing assistive devices and accessories. It also owns Unitron, another hearing aid manufacturer, as well as the cochlear implant manufacturer Advanced Bionics. Sonova also owns Lyric, the extended-wear hearing aid sold under the Phonak brand.

Like many hearing aid manufacturers, Sonova has expanded into the retail business. It owns Hearing Planet, with over 1,600 clinic locations across the country. Sonova recently launched a new global retail chain known as Connect Hearing, and it also entered into a contract with Costco, which sells one of Phonak's premium hearing aids, the Brio, at lower prices than you would get at an independent audiology clinic.

Starkey, a privately held Minnesota-based company, offers a range of hearing aid styles as well as a "not ready for hearing aids" option (hearing amplifiers, discussed in the next chapter). Starkey also has a "made for iPhone" aid, the Halo, which allows signals to stream directly from the phone to your hearing aid.

Starkey hearing aids are sold under differing brand names, including MicroTech, NuEar, Audibel, and AudioSync. Starkey also owns a large retail chain known as Hear Rite.

Widex, based in Denmark, is also a privately held company. Its hearing aid styles have whimsical names like Dream and Passion. Its Mind hearing aid, according to the Widex website, is the first to feature a program dedicated to managing tinnitus, although other manufacturers have followed suit. Widex Baby is, according to the website, the only hearing aid designed specifically for babies, but audiologists say the leading pediatric hearing aids are Phonak BTE's. The Passion is described as "incredibly small," suggesting perhaps that you're more likely to encounter passion if you have an incredibly small hearing aid.

Oticon, a subsidiary of William Demant Holding, celebrated its 110th birthday in 2014. Hans Demant started the company that would become Oticon in 1904 in Odense, Denmark, to help his hearing-impaired wife. Two years earlier, the Danish-born daughter of King Christian IX wore an American-manufactured hearing aid when she married the Prince of Wales, and Oticon lore has it that Hans got the same kind for his wife. As word spread and demand grew, he began selling the American hearing aids, becoming the Danish distributor. During World War II, when importing became difficult, the company began manufacturing them. Oticon, still based in Denmark, is now a global hearing aid and accessories manufacturer. William Demant Holding also owns Bernafon and Sonic Innovations, among others.

Many other smaller hearing aid manufacturers exist. Altogether the various companies offer somewhere around 400 different hearing aids to choose from. Most experts agree that the hearing aids produced by the six largest companies are all good, each boasting slight differences in their technology. The smaller differences lie in fit, appearance, features, accessories, and how the hearing aids work for your particular hearing. The bigger difference will be the result of the skill of the audiologist who programs your hearing aid.

I have had both Widex and Phonak hearing aids. When I got a new hearing aid a few years ago, I went with a Widex, because that was what I'd had before. But I wasn't hearing well with it, so my audiologist ordered a Phonak, which worked better for me. This isn't uncommon: The explanation, my audiologist said, had to do with different algorithms used by different companies. Phonak's happens to suit me better now, though my earlier Widex aid suited me better at that time.

With such slight differences between brands, it's best to consult an audiologist for guidance and recommendations when purchasing a hearing aid.

The Obsession with Invisibility

Many people want the smallest, least visible hearing aid they can get, and companies reinforce this desire through marketing and advertising. "So small they'll never know you're wearing hearing aids!" This kind of sales pitch is annoying to those of us who are trying to promote openness about hearing loss.

That said, most hearing aids *are* invisible these days. Whether behind the ear or in the ear, they are very hard to see, especially on someone with longer hair.

People with cochlear implants are far less sensitive about visibility even though the behind-the-ear device is comparatively huge—as big as a 1950s' hearing aid. In addition it has a wire connecting to a magnet on your head. Women can still conceal it, if they have enough hair, but most people wear their implants proudly. Some even choose vibrant colors or psychedelic patterns.

Hearing aids are already so small that requesting the smallest one you can get is only going to deny you features that will enhance the hearing experience, most notably the telecoil.

The emphasis on invisibility is detrimental to the performance of hearing aids in another way. Hearing aids have come a long way, and the listening experience is far better than it used to be, because of better circuitry. But a smaller device limits the size of these circuits, and the effectiveness of the aid. The smaller hearing aids are recommended only for those with mild to moderately severe hearing loss.

For more serious hearing loss, you'll need a larger hearing aid (though it will still be essentially invisible). Even with the strongest aid, however, there will still be challenges. Although manufacturers may claim clarity of sound for their products, independent studies (and personal experience) show that this is not the case. It is still very hard for those with more severe hearing loss, no matter how good their hearing aids, to hear speech when there is other noise.

And because understanding speech is the reason most people get hearing aids, and because noise is all around us, that is a major issue.

Fine-Tuning Your New Hearing Aid

Your audiologist may have the hearing aids right there, and you can walk out of the store or office with them (on a thirty-, forty-five-, or sixty-day trial basis, typically mandated by state law, with most of the fees refundable). But before you do, the hearing aid will need some fine-tuning to better suit your hearing loss. This is a good reason not to buy them on the Internet, because they rarely come programmed exactly to your specifications, and if they do, it may turn out that your specifications are not exactly what you need.

If your hearing aid is made from a custom mold, it will have to be made at the manufacturer, and it might take a week or two before the finished product arrives at your audiologist's office.

On that visit, the audiologist will fit your new hearing aid into your ear. If it's not comfortable, she may do some minor cosmetic work on it—shaving off a protuberance that seems to be rubbing against the ear, for instance. When it's comfortable, she'll plug a cable into it, connect it to her computer, and run a series of tests to see where the basic factory settings may need adjusting.

Those factory settings, even though they've been tailored to the specifications on your audiogram, probably do need refining. Hearing is a completely subjective experience and what sounds right to one person will not to the next, even if their audiograms are identical.

The audiologist will pull the factory settings up on her screen and try one adjustment after another to make them more appropriate to your hearing loss. My audiologist talks nonstop through this process—but there's a reason for that. As she talks, I hear the changes in the programming. This setting is too tinny, I'll tell her. That one has too much bass. Your voice is loud enough but the words aren't totally clear. At the end of this session, I have a well-tuned hearing aid.

Well-tuned for an audiologist's acoustically perfect office, that is. I always find that when I walk out onto the street, the sounds of real life are a shock. Usually the hearing aids seem to modulate over the next hour or so, although it's actually my brain that is adjusting to the new sound. A good audiologist will have you back for two or more follow-ups for programming, and then see you periodically over the course of the next few months.

Hearing aids contain a lot of complex electronics and they can break down. If your fluctuating hearing persists, you may need the settings reprogrammed. If you gain weight, your hearing aid may feel tight (apparently you can gain weight in your ear), or if you lose weight, the hearing aid may be too loose. You will undoubtedly continue to see your audiologist, for both scheduled and unscheduled visits.

Paying for Your Hearing Aid

Even for the most financially comfortable, six to seven thousand dollars out of pocket for a pair of hearing aids is going make a dent in the bank account. It's wise to insure the hearing aids beyond the two-year warranty.

Children with hearing loss have an easier time getting financial assistance, although it's no guarantee.[30] For adults, the options are very limited. Medicare does not pay for hearing aids, nor do most private insurers. It's worth asking your own carrier, as some may surprise you. Unions may offer a hearing aid credit to cover a portion of the cost. As I mentioned in the introduction, UnitedHealthcare, one of the country's largest insurers, offers affordable hearing aids, beginning at $649, through hi HealthInnovations. AARP offers members hearing aids starting at $795, through HearUSA. Veterans are entitled to hearing aids through Veterans Affairs if the hearing loss is service related. The VA will also pay for batteries. Other options available to veterans can be accessed at the Military Audiology Association website.[31]

In some states, low-income adults may get some reimbursement for hearing aids through Medicaid, though usually only for one ear. Students and some workers may qualify for free hearing aids through their state vocational rehabilitation services. HLAA lists the resources for each state on its website.[32] Some states have hearing aid loan banks, primarily for children.

Audiologists may offer a payment plan that allows the customer to pay for the hearing aids over a period of time. These are similar to dental plans, for instance, that allow payments for major dental work to be spread over the course of one or two years.[33] There are also health-care credit cards that can be used to help finance your hearing aid purchase.

If your employer offers a tax-free health-care spending account, the cost of hearing aids can be paid out of that account. Hearing aids are a federal tax-deductible medical expense. Some but not all states exempt hearing aids and hearing aid batteries from sales tax.

The bottom line is that most people pay for their hearing aids out of pocket. It may be worth discussing the possibility of a discount with your audiologist or hearing aid dealer.

CHAPTER FIVE

The Not-Ready-for-a-Hearing-Aid "Hearing Aid"

Personal Sound Amplification Products.

The Debate over PSAPs

The Food and Drug Administration (FDA) defines a "hearing aid" as "any wearable instrument or device *designed for, offered for the purpose of, or represented as aiding persons with or compensating for impaired hearing*." The FDA defines a PSAP—a Personal Sound Amplification Product—by contrast, as "a wearable electronic product that is not intended to compensate for impaired hearing, but rather is *intended for non-hearing impaired consumers to amplify sounds in certain environments*, such as for hunting or other recreational activities"[34] (italics in both cases are mine). A PSAP cannot be called a hearing aid and cannot be advertised as useful in correcting hearing loss.

The hearing community is divided when it comes to PSAPs.

A hearing aid, as we know, can cost $3,000 or more. A PSAP averages between $100 and $600. Many people think a PSAP, basically a hearing amplifier, is a good alternative to a hearing aid for people with milder hearing loss. So far, the FDA, backed by many professional hearing organizations, does not see it that way. When the FDA proposed tightening restrictions on PSAPs in November 2013, a heated debate took place during the ninety-day comment period that followed.

Those who oppose PSAPs say they are protecting the unwary consumer. As one audiologist commented, "Manufacturers cleverly craft the language of their advertisement to imply that hearing-impaired patients can use PSAPs as inexpensive substitutes for properly fitted hearing aids. Bad experiences with such devices lead patients to conclude that 'hearing aids' don't work."[35] He offered no specifics to back up that claim.

But others—such as the Consumer Electronics Association (which includes among its members most of the PSAP manufacturers)—argued that the low cost gave consumers the opportunity to take the first step toward better hearing. Interestingly, the Hearing Loss Association of America found itself in opposition to its usual allies when it took a neutral stance toward PSAPs: "Consumers say cost is a major barrier to seeking help for their hearing difficulties and purchasing hearing aids. PSAPs might help overcome this obstacle to better hearing."[36] In an interview with the *Hearing Review*, audiologist Patricia Gaffney went further, suggesting that a PSAP "might be a patient's first step toward getting an actual hearing aid."[37]

So how do you know when you need a PSAP versus a hearing aid? Unfortunately, the concept of intended use is another source of debate. In its proposed restrictions, the FDA said that a hearing aid should be used when a person has "difficulty understanding conversations in a crowded room . . . and listening to lectures in an otherwise quiet room." A PSAP, by contrast, should be used when "listening to lectures with a distant speaker . . . distant conversations, performances, etc." In a letter signed by Executive Director Anna Gilmore Hall, the HLAA pointed out the fallacy in this definition: "It's not clear to HLAA what makes the defining difference between a 'lecture with a distant speaker' and 'listening to a lecture in an otherwise quiet room.' At what point is the speaker so far away that a PSAP is acceptable? At what point is a room so quiet that someone who is far away from the speaker needs a hearing aid but not a PSAP?"

As of March 2015, the FDA had issued no new directives on PSAPs.

Then there's the matter of the devices themselves. Are hearing aids and PSAPs really that different? Richard Einhorn doesn't think so. Einhorn is a composer and former classical music producer—someone who, by his description, had "a golden ear." He told me, "I could go into a concert hall, clap my hands, and know whether or not it was appropriate to record classical music." In 2010, he suffered a sudden severe hearing loss. He remains a composer but is now also an advocate for people with hearing loss, an expert on consumer technology for those with hearing loss, and a member of the board of HLAA. In comments he submitted to the FDA, Einhorn listed the essential components of a hearing aid, quoting a major textbook. He went on to note that the same description "also accurately describes products sold as 'personal sound amplifier products,' or 'PSAPs.'" High-quality PSAPs, he continued, are "exactly the same kind of device as a 'hearing aid,' i.e., a miniature public-address system." In an email to me, he added, "The only material difference I'm aware of between them is merely the shape of the container that encloses the electronics." Other experts agree.

I've gone into this discussion at some length because I—and many others—think PSAPs, properly licensed and properly prescribed, could help overturn the resistance to hearing aids. PSAPs remove one of the two major barriers to getting hearing help: cost.

(The second is stigma, and PSAPs are making inroads in that direction as well.)

Buying a PSAP

Consumer Reports cautions that PSAPs "aren't subject to the same safety and effectiveness standards that hearing aids are," and recommends consulting an audiologist before you buy one. Unfortunately, many audiologists at the moment don't want to be consulted about PSAPs. They're in the business of selling hearing aids.

PSAPs are no longer the purview of late-night cable ads, and some are very sophisticated. Major manufacturers have started producing them. Common sense dictates that you not decide on a PSAP until you've had your hearing checked by a professional. But once you know the nature of your loss (seeing an expert to rule out medical conditions that may explain your hearing difficulty), and once you consider and reject the idea of a hearing aid, give the PSAP a try.

PSAPs come in a vast range of brands, prices, styles, and degrees of effectiveness. No one brand dominates the market, and there doesn't seem to be any consumer guide to PSAPs, which is too bad because the offerings are so varied. Most experts advise going for the more expensive devices, which often offer the kind of features found in hearing aids, like ambient noise reduction and Bluetooth connectivity.

Here's a brief overview of some of the PSAPs to choose from, based on my reading of the professional literature (some are footnoted) and interviews with experts on hearing aids and consumer technology. Once again, before purchasing a PSAP it is important to rule out medical conditions that may explain the difficulty hearing you may be having.

Etymotic's Quiet Sound Amplifier, called The Bean, automatically enhances high frequency sounds, which tend to be softer, thus making it easier to understand speech. The Bean, in the shape of a lima bean, fits in the ear and comes in bronze, platinum, or brushed gold. One model includes a telecoil, which works with hearing aid–compatible telephones and loop systems. It also includes a low-battery alert system before the battery dies. The starter package contains a package of batteries and seven ear tips of different sizes for the best possible fit. It uses a #10 battery, which has a nine- to ten-day life, the manufacturer says. It's shipped ready to use, once you insert the battery and fit the ear tip.

In a 2013 blog post on Hearing Health & Technology Matters,[38] Marshall Chasin recommended the Bean for listening to music: "Like the K-AMP of old," he wrote, "the Bean amplifies soft sounds in the higher frequency region but becomes 'acoustically transparent' for louder sounds. It's as if the PSAP pops out of your ear when not needed, and then pops back in only when needed for the softer sounds and harmonics." At the end of February 2015, the Bean was offered on Etymotic's website for $299 each, or $549 for a pair. The T-coil–equipped model is $349, or $599 for a pair. The return policy is thirty days.[39] It can also be purchased online at several sites, including Amazon.com.

Crystal Clear International (CCI)'s Neutronic Ear is also shipped directly to the consumer, ready to use. As of February 2015, the cost from the manufacturer was $499 for one, or $950 for a pair, with a thirty-day trial period. The Neutronic Ear sits in the outer ear (technically, the "bowl of the concha"), leaving the ear canal open to allow natural sound to pass. It, too, includes a low-battery warning and a feedback management system. Two user reviews (both on the manufacturer's website) praised the device for its comfort and clear amplification.

The Sound World Solutions CS50 is a PSAP that can pair with your cell phone via Bluetooth for streaming a variety of audio sources and speaking on the phone. It also, according to the *Hearing Review*, features "improved directionality for listening assistance in noisy environments, such as restaurants." Two rechargeable batteries, which are very easy to connect, come with the device. Each battery takes up to two and a half hours to recharge and reportedly lasts for up to fifteen hours. The CS50 costs $349.99 on Amazon.com or $299 from Sound World Solutions directly.

Able Planet, a Colorado headphone manufacturer, makes a dozen or so PSAPs in a variety of styles and colors. Some are worn in the ear and others behind the ear. Like many PSAPs, they are designed to enhance sound in noisy environments and also include a feedback manager. The more expensive cost about $475. Like many of these devices, they may employ sophisticated technology, such as multichannel signals and sometimes Bluetooth connectivity.[40]

One of the most promising PSAPs is the Soundhawk Smart Listening System, made by a company of the same name based in Cupertino, California, high-tech heaven. The three-part system includes the earpiece (or "scoop"), a wireless microphone, and a free smartphone app. According to David Kirkwood, of Hearing Health & Technology Matters, "The patented app uses dozens of algorithms to filter, mute, amplify or otherwise alter sound." The user moves a finger across the smartphone screen to adjust the volume. The scoop is designed to enhance certain frequencies and reduce background noise. Among its features is the microphone clip, which a speaker can wear in a restaurant or other noisy place. The voice is transmitted without ambient-noise interference to the scoop and from there to the cochlea and brain.

The Soundhawk came on the market in November 2014, at $300, and received a favorable review from *The New York Times*'s tech columnist Farhad Manjoo.[41] Manjoo noted that the Soundhawk "was designed by audio scientists who have worked at some of the world's best hearing-aid companies. The company has also hired alumni from Apple, Amazon, and other tech hardware companies to make its device both stylish and easy to use." For years, people have complained about poor design and performance in hearing devices, and lamented the need for a Steve Jobs of hearing loss. Soundhawk is not for everyone—certainly not for someone with severe hearing loss, like me—but it is a viable alternative for many with mild to moderate loss not yet willing to commit to hearing aids.

While it may have a sleek design, the Soundhawk is a very visible device. It looks just like a Bluetooth headset. Everyone wants invisible hearing aids, but they're perfectly happy to walk around with something that looks like a big Bluetooth headset attached to their ear.

I am not recommending any one of these devices, nor do hearing experts who have written about them. The choice is personal, and should in part be dictated by advice from a professional—an audiologist, if you can find one who will discuss PSAPs. The prices seem to change with some frequency, and many of them had dropped during the period between the time I first wrote this chapter and when it was fact-checked a few months later. This is a new field, and for now the consumer will be hard-pressed to find a guide.

Promoters of these devices take pains to say that they are not substitutes for hearing aids. Soundhawk's CEO, Michael Kisch, says the device is intended for use in specific situations, like a restaurant. The company anticipates a consumer would use it for only two to four hours a day (a statement that may be for the benefit of the FDA, because any claim that it works like a hearing aid is illegal).

PSAP advocates like to think of these as starter devices. They say that if an audiologist recommends the product to someone who is not ready for a hearing aid, two or three years later that customer may come back ready to plunk down $3,000–$4,000 for the real thing.

I don't want to end this chapter without mentioning Williams Sound's venerable "Pocketalker," a handheld amplifier with a microphone, about the size of a deck of cards, attached to headphones for the person who needs to hear better. The cost is less than $200. You can buy it at Amazon, among other retailers. Because the

Pocketalker is not attuned to your specific hearing, it can be used by anyone right out of the box. Make sure you set the volume low at first.

Barbara Weinstein, founding executive officer of the Doctor of Audiology program at the City University of New York and an advocate for hearing devices for the elderly, says the Pocketalker "truly can make a difference in the lives of people with significant hearing loss who need to communicate but are not ready for or are not candidates for hearing aids or PSAPs."

Some nursing homes or rehab facilities keep them on hand for short-term use by patients with hearing loss, as does the VA Hospital in New York. Pocket talkers are "very helpful on a short-term basis for seniors who are having difficulty hearing in a one-on-one situation," Kassie Witte, coordinator of audiology at the Hebrew Home at Riverdale in the Bronx, told a columnist for *The New York Times*'s New Old Age blog.[42]

Weinstein adds: "In my ideal world, every nursing home and assisted living facility would have these devices available on the floor for visitors to use to communicate with residents." They would also be useful in hospital emergency rooms.

The Future of PSAPs

You can buy a PSAP for $20 or $30, but they probably won't be worth what you spent on them. The higher-quality products, however, do seem like a viable substitute for hearing aids for those who cannot afford hearing aids, or aren't ready for them. When I first started writing about hearing loss, in 2010, PSAPs were clunky, unreliable devices you might buy on the Internet or by mail order. Today, just five years later, we're seeing the beginning of a revolution in attitudes toward the treatment of hearing loss.

As long as Medicare refuses to reimburse for hearing aids, as long as audiologists charge $3,000 to $4,000 for products that have to be supplemented by other products that cost another $1,000, as long as the lifespan of a hearing aid is about five years (meaning another huge investment), people with mild loss are going to look elsewhere for hearing help for as long as they possibly can. Eventually, they may need a real hearing aid. But Personal Sound Amplification Products will allow them to go on hearing and participating in life until then.

In a 2014 keynote address to the Academy of Doctors of Audiology, Dr. Frank Lin, one of the most widely respected researchers in the area of hearing loss and cognition, detoured from his stated topic to discuss the use of PSAPs. "The air became a bit chillier," an article in the *Hearing Review* noted, as Dr. Lin described PSAPs "as good low-cost solutions for the hearing impaired population." He told the audience that his group was researching the use of a self-programmable device (the Sound World Solutions CS50, mentioned earlier in this chapter) using community health-care workers for screening, education, and monitoring. Acknowledging that hearing aids dispensed by audiologists are the "gold standard," he added that they will not be widely used until they're covered by Medicare.

I hope audiologists will embrace PSAPs, so that if we buy them, we can be sure we are getting the right hearing device for us. I hope the FDA will regulate them for safety and effectiveness. I hope that acceptance of PSAPs by hearing professionals will ensure that anyone purchasing one will have had their hearing checked to make sure there are no underlying causes of their hearing loss. But until these changes happen, the market will continue to expand without the guidance, oversight, and protection that independent audiologists and FDA regulation would provide.

CHAPTER SIX

How Did This Happen?

For many people the most frustrating part of hearing loss is not knowing the cause.

I lost most of my hearing between the ages of thirty and sixty, and doctors still don't have a clue as to the cause. For a long time, I was incredulous that there was no diagnosis, but now I understand how often this is true, especially with hearing loss that has a sudden onset. The lack of an explanation was especially distressing because if my doctors had been able to pinpoint a cause, they might have prevented the continuing deterioration. Maybe I would not now be profoundly deaf in my left ear and with serious hearing loss in the right.

Why is it so difficult to pinpoint the cause of hearing loss? Sometimes it's a lot easier to measure the degree of the loss than it is to determine how it happened. Many factors affect hearing and cause hearing loss, and causes may overlap or may not be apparent at all. In this chapter, I will discuss some of the causes of adult-onset hearing loss, leaving childhood deafness to others.

Adult-onset hearing loss has not received as much research attention as childhood deafness, in part because of the same stigma that has kept so many from treating their loss. "Hearing loss is often treated as an unavoidable and relatively unimportant consequence of aging," Johns Hopkins's Dr. Frank Lin said at a 2014 symposium on hearing loss and healthy aging.[43] "Yet it clearly contributes to a variety of physical, cognitive, and psychological problems."

Dr. Lin pointed out that this attitude doesn't just apply to those with hearing loss: Researchers and hearing health providers also tend to dismiss hearing loss as a natural and insignificant consequence of aging. The result is that it has been hard to get research grants for something as mundane as age-related hearing loss. That is changing, as we begin to realize not only that hearing loss affects many people well before old age, but also that the cost of untreated hearing loss is immense both personally and in terms of public health dollars.

Noise

The most common causes of hearing loss are aging and noise. The danger from noise is a function of exposure time plus intensity. The louder the noise, the shorter the period of time you can safely be exposed to it.

When that child behind you on the airplane shrieks from New York to L.A., you may worry for your hearing. But it's probably not doing permanent damage. It's only a five-hour flight and even the most persistent shrieker can't maintain a damaging decibel level for that amount of time.

The plane itself is loud of course. This is probably a bigger problem for flight attendants than passengers, who have much briefer exposures and can also wear headphones. Noise inside the plane

How loud is too loud?

The noise chart below lists average decibel levels for everyday sounds around you.

PAINFUL

150 dB = fireworks at 3 feet

140 dB = firearms, jet engine

130 dB = jackhammer

120 dB = jet plane takeoff, siren

EXTREMELY LOUD

110 dB = maximum output of some MP3 players, model airplane, chain saw

106 dB = gas lawn mower, snowblower

100 dB = hand drill, pneumatic drill

90 dB = subway, passing motorcycle

VERY LOUD

80–90 dB = blow-dryer, kitchen blender, food processor

70 dB = busy traffic, vacuum cleaner, alarm clock

MODERATE

60 dB = typical conversation, dishwasher, clothes dryer

50 dB = moderate rainfall

40 dB = quiet room

FAINT

30 dB = whisper, quiet library

during takeoff and landing can reach 105 decibels, according the American Speech-Language-Hearing Association.[44] Cruising sound level is usually around 85 decibels, though the noise can be louder in the back of the plane. On short-hop flights, airlines often still use propeller planes, which are very very loud.

Far more dangerous is regular exposure. We regulate it (pretty well) in the workplace, but leisure activities are often literally deafening. Sports is one of the worst offenders: Teams celebrate "the twelfth man"—noise—and vie to break decibel-level records. Stadiums can easily reach 130 decibels. That's going to cause some permanent damage. The noise at Seattle's Century Link Field was measured at 137.6 in December 2013, which set off a minor earthquake.[45] Subway noise, construction noise, music at rock concerts and parties, and listening on your personal devices can all contribute to hearing loss over time.

The American Speech-Language-Hearing Association offers an easy-to-read chart on common noise levels, which I have reprinted here. You can find it at asha.org/public/hearing/Noise/.

The louder the noise, the shorter the time you should be exposed to it. Anyone using a lawnmower, snow blower, leaf blower, or chainsaw regularly should wear noise-canceling headphones.

Noise levels outside the workplace are rarely monitored or regulated. We expose ourselves to damaging noise in leisure activities every single day. From restaurants to sports stadiums to our own backyards, dangerous levels of noise are a feature of daily life. The noise begins at a young age: Many toys intended for toddlers exceed recommended noise levels.[46]

By the time you're old enough for age-related hearing loss, at seventy or so, you are probably already suffering from noise-related hearing loss. Determining if hearing loss is due to noise or age is difficult. While the physiologic changes in the ear differ, the hearing loss often looks similar on an audiogram. Both types are bilateral (unless the noise exposure was a sudden loud sound close to one ear), affect the high frequencies, and are gradual in onset, and the loss is generally the same in both ears.

What about those ear buds? iPods and other MP3 players are a highly visible example of noise exposure. If someone is wearing in-the-ear buds twelve hours a day to screen out other loud noise, it's probably doing damage. Newer ear buds have maximum settings, so if you're worried about a teenager, buy him a fancy new set of ear buds with a noise cap. You can also set the cap on a smartphone. (Just don't tell him why.) Try to minimize listening to music while jogging or doing other vigorous exercise, where you'll be tempted to turn it up, especially if you already have a hearing loss. There are exceptions, of course, from something as unexpected as a malfunctioning cell phone that emits a piercing sound in the user's ear to the damage done by an explosive device, which may affect just one ear or both.

Noise-related hearing loss is a major problem in the military. More disability claims are made for hearing loss and tinnitus (from service-related incidents) than any other categories. They may accompany traumatic brain injury or post-traumatic stress disorder but more often occur on their own.[47] In 2010, hearing-related disability claims stemming from the global war on terror were estimated at nearly 300,000. Total hearing-related claims (from all wars) were more than 1.5 million.

Factory workers, miners, farmers, construction workers, road crews, etc., all simply accept that the job will eventually affect their hearing. When I started working at the *Times* in the late 1980s, the press rooms were still in the basement. When the presses were running, you couldn't hear over the din. A hearing test was part of the hiring process. If an employee later filed a workmen's compensation suit, claiming that workplace noise had injured his hearing, the *Times* would have a record of what it had been when the employee was hired. The *Times* employed several Deaf workers in the press rooms, avoiding the problem of noise exposure damage.

In 1970, President Richard Nixon signed the Occupational Safety and Health Act, with bipartisan congressional backing—despite opposition from businesses. The operation arm was OSHA, the Occupational Safety and Health Administration. OSHA protects workers in most nongovernmental workplaces that are not covered by other agencies (for instance, by the Federal Aviation Administration or the Mine Safety and Health Administration). The act also created NIOSH, the National Institute for Occupational Safety and Health, as a research agency.

The loudest industries today are not the ones you might initially think of: At the top of the list, according to OSHA, are those that employ meat packers, followed by textile and leather workers, lumber workers and machine feeders in the furniture and fixtures industry, and paper products workers. OSHA doesn't represent rock bands, professional football teams, or dance club employees, all of whom probably measure right up there with meat packers.

OSHA's regulations are often disputed because they're based not just on the noise level in the workplace but exposure over time, which is complicated to assess when workers move from one area to another or do different kinds of work on a single shift.

When OSHA was set up in 1971, regulations allowed workers to be exposed to 90 decibels for a maximum of eight hours, and 100 decibels for a maximum of two. These caps still exist today. Many people think this is too loud for too long. NIOSH recommends exposure to 100 decibels for no more than 15 minutes (total, not continuous) per day of exposure, or else the worker runs the risk of permanent hearing damage.

The more heated controversy comes with industry's approach to compliance. Although OSHA sets these noise levels, it does not require employers to correct them through administrative or engineering controls (for instance, moving affected workers to quieter areas or installing noise abatement structures) until noise exposures reach 100 decibels over eight hours, and only then if the controls are "feasible."

Up until that point, employers can simply give workers earmuffs or earplugs. OSHA sets the rules for permissible exposure, but the Department of Labor is responsible for enforcing them. The employer is required to provide hearing protection but the employee is not required to wear them. Until recently the older model of ear protection often prevented wearers from hearing sounds they needed to hear, like other workers or even alarms.

Aging

As they say, it's better than the alternative. Even though I like to remind people that more than half of those with hearing loss in this country are under the age of fifty-five, it is also a fact that hearing declines with aging. It's not inevitable—my mother heard perfectly until she was almost ninety—but it is very likely. Ninety percent of those over eighty have "clinically significant"[48] hearing loss, and of that group 80 percent have severe enough loss that they would benefit from hearing aids (only 15 percent of this group has hearing aids).

As long as we are talking numbers here, it's important to note how many of those 48 million Americans are seriously affected by their hearing loss. According to the NIDCD, about 2 percent of adults aged forty-five to fifty-four have disabling hearing loss. The rate increases to 8.5 percent for adults aged fifty-five to sixty-four. Nearly 25 percent of those aged sixty-five to seventy-four and 50 percent of those who are seventy-five and older have disabling hearing loss.[49]

Both noise- and age-related hearing loss are sensorineural, meaning that the hair cells of the inner ears are no longer able to propel sound to the auditory nerve for passage to the brain. Noise-related loss is thought to accelerate hearing loss from aging. Noise kills some hair cells outright. But it may just damage others, leaving them vulnerable to other assaults later on, for instance from age. If you can protect your hearing when you're young, you have a better chance of avoiding debilitating hearing loss in old age.

Genes

Genetic, or hereditary, hearing loss, accounts for about 60 percent of deafness in infants. Though they have inherited the genetic defect, it does not mean they are born to deaf parents. Nine out of ten deaf children are born to hearing parents. In about 70 percent of cases of genetic loss, it is "non-syndromic," that is, it isn't associated with any other clinical abnormalities. The genetic defect may skip generations, and often the parents will not be aware of hearing loss in their families, although researchers can often trace a genetic pattern. Fifteen to 30 percent of hereditary deafness is associated with other abnormalities—like Usher syndrome, which causes both blindness and deafness—ranging from mild to severe.[50]

Researchers think it's likely that genetics also plays a role in deafness in the elderly, especially among women. Anecdotally, this makes sense: Some people work in noisy environments their whole life and never suffer hearing loss. Some people also smoke and never get lung cancer. The reverse is true as well: People who spend their lives in bucolic peace lose their hearing, and nonsmokers get lung cancer. We don't know why this is in either case but it probably comes down to genetics. Otolaryngologists like to talk about tough ears—ears that are resistant to damage. They can't pinpoint the gene for toughness, but it's there.

They *can* pinpoint some of the genes associated with hereditary hearing loss. In some families, hereditary loss follows a consistent pattern. The women in the family, for instance, all begin to lose their hearing at about the same age. One friend of mine began to lose her hearing at thirty-five, as had her mother and grandmother. Researchers looking for a biological cure for hearing loss, through gene therapy or stem cell therapy, think that they'll find a cure for—or more likely a way to prevent—genetic hearing loss sooner than other kinds of loss. Several labs are very close to making gene-therapy treatments a clinical reality.

Ototoxic Drugs and Chemicals

The word *ototoxin* literally means "hearing poison." Ototoxins include common prescription and nonprescription drugs, ranging from the seemingly benign, like aspirin and ibuprofen, to powerful chemotherapy drugs. People with hereditary loss may be more susceptible to their effects.

Overreliance on antibiotics is harmful to your health on many levels, including your hearing health. Aminoglycoside antibiotics (gentamicin, streptomycin, and others) cause hearing loss, in large enough doses and especially when combined with other drugs like vancomycin or a loop diuretic. So can the fluoroquinolones, including Cipro and Levaquin.

Antidepressants—including Prozac, Elavil, Paxil, Zoloft, and Celexa —have been linked to tinnitus. (They are also often prescribed to relieve the psychological burden of tinnitus.) Loop diuretics (like Lasix), prescribed for heart or kidney problems, can affect metabolic activity in the inner ear, contributing to hearing loss.

Among the most predictably damaging drugs are cisplatin and its relative, carboplatin, both common chemotherapy drugs. If you know you have a family history of hearing loss, or have begun to experience it for other reasons, oncologists may suggest substituting other drugs for chemotherapy. But if it's a case of your life or your hearing, most people will feel there's no choice.

Drugs like aspirin, quinine (for treatment of malaria), and loop diuretics require much larger doses and longer-term use than some of the others before they have an effect on hearing, and the hearing loss can often be reversed if you stop taking them.

In general, if you take daily multiple doses of any of these drugs and notice some hearing loss, the drug may be the cause. They affect the cochlear hair cells, damaging hearing, but they are rarely toxic to the vestibular system as a whole. Therefore, most researchers think they do not cause Ménière's disease, BPPV (benign paroxysmal positional vertigo), or other kinds of vertigo. They may well cause tinnitus. Some of the aminoglycosides are toxic to the balance system and hearing.

Environmental toxins can also damage hearing. Exposure to mercury can lead to permanent hearing and balance problems. Other environmental chemicals that damage hearing include butyl nitrite, carbon disulfide, styrene, carbon monoxide, tin, hexane, toluene, lead, trichloroethylene, manganese, and xylene. These are all hazardous to much more than your hearing, and are mainly encountered in industrial professions. Butyl nitrite is recreationally used as poppers.

Disease

Some diseases that make you sick also damage your hearing. Bacterial infections are a major cause of childhood hearing loss, especially in developing countries where vaccines may be scarce. Measles, mumps, and meningitis may all cause permanent hearing loss. (These diseases can also affect adults, with the same result, but they're rarer in adults.)

Chronic or untreated ear infections, called otitis media, affect the middle ear. Sometimes chronic otitis media can result in cholesteatoma, a mass of cells that grows into a tumor in the middle ear and blocks hearing.

Bacterial meningitis and the antibiotics used to treat it can affect the hearing of adults or children who survive this often deadly disease. Helen Keller lost both her sight and hearing after she developed a high fever at the age of nineteen months, which experts believe was caused by scarlet fever or meningitis. Prompt treatment with powerful antibiotics can sometimes reverse meningitis, but both the meningitis and the antibiotics can leave survivors with temporary, but more often permanent hearing loss. Cochlear implant surgery has very occasionally resulted in cases of meningitis, and for that reason a meningitis vaccine is required before the surgery.

Otosclerosis, a disease of the bones of the middle ear, is most prevalent in adults, particularly Caucasians. The National Institute on Deafness and Other Communication Disorders reports that otosclerosis affects three million Americans, with white middle-aged women at highest risk. The condition is less common in people of Japanese and South American decent and is rare in African Americans. (Age-related hearing loss is also rarer in dark-skinned people, according to some studies.) Even if you fit none of these higher-risk categories, you're not immune. Otosclerosis can be seen in any person, at any age.

The hallmark symptom of otosclerosis, slowly progressing hearing loss, usually starts in the early twenties. Over the ensuing several years, the hearing loss becomes more significant. Otosclerosis affects one ear at first, and often the second ear. Approximately 60 percent of cases are genetic in origin. On average, a person who has one parent with otosclerosis has a 25 percent chance of developing the disorder. If both parents have it, the risk goes up to 50 percent. Interestingly, pregnancy can be a trigger for hearing loss associated with otosclerosis. Rubella virus has been implicated in some cases of otosclerosis, as well.[51]

Sudden Hearing Loss

If you find that you've lost your hearing overnight, or over the course of a few days, whether in one ear or both, you should go straight to an ENT, or an emergency room, as quickly as possible. (If you go to the ER, be sure to ask for an ENT doctor.)

Sudden hearing loss is a medical emergency and should be treated within the first two weeks of onset. "Sudden hearing loss" is not just a description—it's a diagnosis. It means you have lost 30 decibels of hearing—a substantial amount—over three contiguous frequencies in less than three days, a pattern that is readily apparent on an audiogram. If you've never had an audiogram and there is no reference point, the audiologist uses the undamaged ear for reference. It usually occurs in just one ear and it is always caused by damage to the hair cells in the inner ear or by nerve damage. [52]

It's an unpredictable condition, and most cases are idiopathic, caused by vascular, viral, or some combination of factors. Sometimes it resolves itself over the following days or weeks. But if it doesn't, and if it hasn't been treated, it will likely become permanent. A physician should refer anyone with sudden hearing loss to an ENT immediately. The ENT will order a series of tests, including an MRI to rule out a tumor on the auditory nerve. He will also start the patient on a course of steroids, either in pill form or through the eardrum. The full steroid course takes two weeks, at which point you go back to the doctor for a follow-up visit.

Steroids are powerful drugs and taking them for something that may reverse itself naturally may seem like overkill. But if the hearing loss doesn't reverse itself, you've lost the two-week window in which treatment with steroids is most effective. Most ENTs treat sudden hearing loss with steroids immediately, before they get the results of an MRI or blood tests back.

If your hearing loss remains at the new lower level, and no underlying causes have been found, you will be diagnosed with sudden hearing loss. Recommendations for treatment vary. Until very recently, the most common were CROS or BiCROS hearing aids, which are worn on the bad ear and transmit sound to the good ear wirelessly. CROS hearing aids are used in single-sided deafness (SSD) when the good ear is normal. BiCROS are used when the better ear has some moderate loss. Some experts feel these devices have been superseded by technology that programs a regular hearing aid to transmit sound wirelessly to a hearing aid on the non-hearing side.[53] Others, like audiologist Barbara Weinstein, think the CROS and BiCROS have benefited from advances in digital technology and should still be considered for these cases.

Some conditions are initially diagnosed as sudden hearing loss but if the degree or nature of the loss changes, so does the diagnosis.

If the hearing fluctuates, and if it's accompanied by fullness in the ear, dizziness, or tinnitus, you may be diagnosed with Ménière's Disease, which is an imbalance of the fluids in the inner ear. Ménière's itself may be idiopathic—having no known cause.

If it turns out that your hearing has continued to drop despite the steroids, it could be a rare condition called AIED (Autoimmune Inner Ear Disease).

According to the NIDCD, in only 10 to 15 percent of people diagnosed with sudden hearing loss is there an identifiable cause.

Often after the initial diagnosis of sudden hearing loss, the hearing, and thus the diagnosis, changes. That's what happened to me. In my case, it changed to idiopathic, cause unknown.

Sudden hearing loss is a relatively rare condition. I'm giving it this space because it is a serious kind of loss that can sometimes be reversed—but only if you act quickly enough. Because the symptoms resemble a cold or congestion, most people don't seek medical help immediately. Even if they call their primary care physician, they'll probably be told to try decongestants. Meanwhile, the clock is ticking. By the time they finally get to the ENT, it's too late to treat. If your hearing is noticeably diminished and you are concerned about sudden hearing loss even if your primary care physician isn't, don't wait: Find an ENT.

CHAPTER SEVEN

Practice, Practice, Practice

Getting used to hearing aids is not a passive act.

You've been to the audiologist; you've got your hearing aid; you've paid top dollar for it. It can be a rude shock to find out that you still can't understand what people are saying.

Why can't a hearing aid be more like glasses? I still remember the day when I was six years old and saw treetops for the first time. I walked into the optometrist with fuzzy vision and walked out with 20/20 perfection.

Hearing aids often take more work.

Many factors influence the perception of success with a new hearing aid. Some of them are objective, having to do with the technology. Some are subjective, having to do with the individual's expectations and degree of hearing loss.

A Negative Attitude Usually Means a Negative Outcome

The person who gets the hearing aids has to want them. If you tell your mother she really should get hearing aids, and she reluctantly goes along with the plan to humor you or get you off her back, she probably won't like them. And if she doesn't like them, they'll end up in the drawer.

Remember Dr. Powers and his diagnosis of "GOMD"—grumpy old man disease? That guy is not going to get a hearing aid if he has anything to do with it, and if he does, he's not going to wear it. Even if he agrees to try it, his attitude will be so dismissive that there's no way he'll ever see the benefit.

A reluctant senior might not like the hearing aids you've gone out and gotten for her for a variety of reasons. If she hasn't participated in the fitting and adjusting with an open mind, she's probably going home with hearing aids that aren't working very well. She may find it uncomfortable to wear something in her ear. If the hearing aid is too loose, it may squeal. If it's too tight, it will hurt. If she can't manipulate the hearing aid herself—because her fingers are arthritic or the hearing aid is small—she'll feel it's yet another thing she doesn't have any control over.

Most of all, though, after years of what was probably gradually increasing hearing loss, it can be a shock to hear again. The world is loud and most hearing aids amplify fairly indiscriminately. They may sound okay in the audiologist's office, but the minute the wearer walks out into real life she'll feel assaulted by noise. By street noise, by the clatter of dishes or the roar of a vacuum cleaner, by the babel of voices she's suddenly hearing.

This is why counseling is so important when getting a hearing aid. The potential user has to understand the benefits, but he also has to understand that the device may not restore perfect hearing—at least not the first time out. Realistic expectations are critical to satisfaction.

If your mother is reluctant to get hearing aids, you have to suggest some concrete benefits: She'll be able to understand her grandchildren. She'll be able to talk on the phone with you after you go home, across the country. She'll be able to hear the numbers called out at bingo, go to concerts, hear her partner's bid at the bridge table, audit a class at a nearby university. Even mild to moderate hearing loss makes many of these things impossible. And that's the degree of hearing loss that hearing aids are most successful in correcting.

Journalist Margery D. Rosen had some other good suggestions in a column she wrote recently for AARP.[54] One of the best, I thought, was to introduce your reluctant loved one to someone who does well with hearing aids. Find a good role model. She also suggests encouraging the reluctant user just to try it. Hearing aid manufacturers allow you to test products, for from thirty to sixty days, depending on the manufacturer and state laws.

But it was Rosen's last suggestion that surprised me with its astuteness. Stop being an enabler: "You've probably been repeating and explaining things for so long that you don't even realize you've become an enabler, acting as your loved one's personal hearing device," she wrote. "Unfortunately, this just causes your loved one to continue to put off needed treatment."

You could also mention cognitive decline. The person who needs the hearing aids probably takes vitamins and cholesterol medication and maybe blood pressure medication. In the same way these are preventive—keeping your cholesterol or blood pressure low enough to avoid strokes and heart attacks—so are hearing aids, in keeping the mind active to help avoid cognitive decline. Moreover, some evidence suggests that wearing a hearing aid can prevent further reduction in speech understanding.[55]

The issues are slightly different with reluctant younger people. The stigma of age is powerful, and so is the fear of discrimination in the workplace. It may be hard to persuade a younger person that hearing aids are in her own best interest.

News stories confirm that concern. A few years ago, two New York City police officers, both with more than twenty years of service, were forced to retire when the department decided to enforce a policy on hearing aids. Even though the NYPD had paid for the hearing aids, and the officers had been wearing them for some time, they were now told to pack up and take their pensions. Police regulations, they were told, forbade them to take the NYPD hearing test wearing hearing aids. The officers sued the City of New York and the NYPD, and in March 2015 the case was settled in their favor. Under the terms of the settlement, the NYPD must allow any officers who request hearing aids to take the standard NYPD hearing test *wearing* their hearing aids. Their ability to perform "essential functions" will be considered on a case-by-case basis, with evaluation of the specific job tasks taken into consideration.

No one wants police officers who can't hear. But NYPD's blanket policy was a clear violation of the Americans with Disabilities Act (ADA). As Stuart Seaborn of Disability Rights Advocates, told me, "What's really a precedent is the decision to consider hearing loss on a case-by-case analysis." He and others acknowledge that some hearing loss is not fully correctable. "There is some hearing loss that is so severe that it's not appropriate for police work. We don't want a blanket ruling either way. We want evaluation of what someone can do on a case-by-case basis."[56]

For most people in the workplace, a hearing aid is in no way a deterrent to job performance. For people with mild to moderate loss, a hearing aid can restore lost functions, make it easier to join in conversations, and make being with friends and family more enjoyable.

Set Yourself Up for Success

Expectations affect success with hearing aids. If they're too high, you'll be disappointed. If they're too low, you may give up before you get started. You'll never do the sustained wearing that allows your ears and brain to adjust to the hearing aid. Expectations have to be just right.

Appropriate choice of hearing aids also affects success. That's why the audiologist should ask the client questions before he or she decides to get a hearing aid or chooses a type. More features are not necessarily better. More expensive is not necessarily better. For some people the most basic hearing aids will be much easier to deal with, and will thus be used. For others, more sophisticated technology may make them feel more confident about the hearing aid.

Acceptance of the hearing loss also affects outcome. People who are still in denial are not going to get much benefit from hearing aids because they don't think they need them, don't want them, don't want other people to know they have them. That's a recipe for failure.

Adjusting to a New Hearing Aid

It's a little like ordering a table from IKEA: When it arrives in that flat box with a little plastic bag full of nuts and bolts and assembly directions, you still have a lot of work to do before you can eat dinner on it.

The hearing aid or aids do arrive assembled, no nuts or bolts included, but they may not sound right at first.

The factory settings are based on the tests the audiologist did the first time around, including the audiogram and other tests. Factory settings are not usually optimal, however, because hearing is a subjective sense. Audiometrics (numbers) are not the only answer. What's music to my ears is noise to yours.

The audiologist will plug your new hearing aid into her

computer and adjust the programming while asking you a stream of questions. How does this sound? Is it too loud? How does my voice sound? How does your own voice sound? All the while she's fiddling with the dials on the computer, taking into account your responses.

Even if the factory settings are right for you, they'll take time to get used to. For instance, if you have high frequency loss, what you hear through the hearing aid may sound tinny or harsh once those high frequencies are restored. The audiologist may suggest you set the volume lower as you adjust to the new high frequency sounds. The audiological consensus is that within a month of sustained hearing aid use, you will have adjusted to the new sounds.

Unfortunately, that's also approaching the time limit for return or exchange without penalty. So if you suspect you're not making progress, don't wait until the end of a month to go back to the audiologist. You may well need to try a different hearing aid. Over the years, I've gotten four new hearing aids. Not once has the initial try been correct. Sometimes I've gone through three or four brands or styles before I find the one that seems best for me, leaving custom-made ear molds in my wake.

It's not just your ears that are adjusting, but also your brain. Your brain has adapted to not hearing certain sounds. It has to readapt once they're reintroduced.

Most startling is the sound of your own voice. *Who is that?* I always think when I get a new hearing aid and hear myself talk. If you have a hearing aid that fills the ear canal, it's plugging your ears—though a vent in the hearing aid should minimize this effect. Again, it may take several weeks of sustained hearing aid use for your voice to sound like you.

Sustained Use Is Key

Most audiologists recommend wearing new hearing aids all the time, to expedite adapting to them. If you're not comfortable with that, start with at least three or four hours a day and gradually increase the time. The more you wear your hearing aids, the better they will sound and the quicker the adjustment time.

Once you've adjusted to the initial settings, however, you can probably tolerate even more sound from the hearing aid. That's why follow-up visits every few weeks in the early months are important. Your initial setting is probably not the maximal setting for you. But if you started out with the maximal setting you wouldn't be able to tolerate it.

Even once you have acclimated yourself to the hearing aid, you may still need more hearing help. The sad fact is, as one recent article noted, "Amplification alone most often falls short in fully addressing all of the daily communication challenges the adult with hearing loss confronts in the home, at work, and within the larger milieu of society."[57]

This may mean you need to buy additional equipment, which I'll discuss in Chapter 18. But you can also teach your ears—and your brain—to hear better with those new hearing aids.

Train Your Brain

The majority of people will hear much better if they take advantage of auditory rehab programs. These may be offered through your audiologist but you can also find them at community health centers, at hearing centers like the Center for Hearing and Communication[58] in New York and Florida, and online.

Hearing rehab can be done at home on your own. Even something as simple as listening to a recorded book and then checking against the text is good training. Your brain needs to learn how to hear again, and that comes with practice.

The speech pathways in the brain get rusty with disuse. (Not literally, of course. What actually happens is that the pathways get taken over by other senses, primarily vision, in a process called "cross-modal plasticity.") You can retrain them to hear, and you can keep them active by wearing your hearing aids all the time, by listening supplemented by reading captions, by talking on the telephone rather than emailing.

Quite a few programs can be found online. They are designed for recipients of cochlear implants, which I'll describe in Chapter 21, but they can also be useful for new hearing aid users. Other programs, like Angel Sound,[59] developed by researchers at the House Research Institute in California, are good for hearing aid or cochlear implant users. Beware, though, that some of these programs can be downloaded only onto PCs, not on Apple computers except by first downloading some translational software.

The LACE program (Listening and Communication Enhancement[60]), which was developed by two UCSF audiologists, is available in three increasingly sophisticated levels, with programs for both PC and Mac, as well as on DVD. The prices increase with the level. LACE training is intensive and requires commitment from the trainee, optimally five days a week, thirty minutes per session. The training exposes the listener to speech in noise, gradually increasing the ratio of noise to speech. It teaches you how to focus on one speaker when others are talking, how to supply the one word in a sentence you may have missed, speech-reading, and general strategies for maximizing your hearing. It's similar to clinician-based programs, but it's done at home. It can go on for as long or short a time as you wish and feel you are benefiting from it.

If your audiologist doesn't suggest auditory therapy in either a formal program or one of the at-home programs, ask about it. Even if your audiologist forgets to suggest you wear the hearing aid all day every day, do it. It's the only way you'll get the fullest possible benefit.

Practice is essential. Still, if you find you simply can't improve much with those hearing aids or a cochlear implant, don't blame yourself. Although researchers agree that a hearing aid user can better their chances of success with practice, they also agree that outcomes are unpredictable. So do whatever you can to give yourself the best possible chance at hearing well with the hearing aids. And if that doesn't work, you may want to consider assistive devices, the subject of Chapter 18.

But before we move on to more technology, I want to address some of the issues that people with hearing loss face in their everyday lives, with or without hearing aids.

PART TWO

Love
and Work

CHAPTER EIGHT

Family Matters

*Spouses, children, grandparents—hearing loss
is a family affair.*

Paradoxically, it may be within the comfort of home that one is most aware of the effects of hearing loss. For most of us, it's the place where we let our guard down and relax. It's also the place where people—people who love us!—feel most free to confront us about denial, about getting our hearing treated. And it's where the pain of our loss can feel most acute.

Whether the hearing loss is recent and still relatively mild or established and fairly severe, it really is a family affair. A study by a British hearing group on the impact of hearing loss on family noted that while it is typically considered at an individual level—with diagnosis and treatment impacting only the affected person—the experience of hearing loss is shared, and managed, by the person's spouse or partner and other family members.[61]

Here's to the Long-Suffering Spouse!

Being hard of hearing can make you testy. You get tired of saying *What?* all the time. You get tired of your spouse tossing off remarks as he walks out of the room. You get tired of him shouting something at you from the living room when you're in the kitchen. Et cetera, et cetera. Those et ceteras could go on for paragraphs.

But being married to someone with hearing loss can make the hearing spouse testy. And this is when you're married to someone who *admits* to hearing loss. Being married to someone who says everything's fine, it's *your* fault for mumbling, is something else altogether.

Woe to my husband in those dark years as my hearing plunged inexorably. Luckily, he is still married to me, and no longer in woe. But I was a terror. I was desperately unhappy about the loss, fearful and anxious about my job, worried that people would find out, furious at everyone and everything. I simmered with anger at the dinner table as my family talked over and around me. Sometimes I slammed my hand down on the table and said I couldn't understand a word. Then often I'd burst into tears and stomp out of the room, slamming the door behind me. This was a family, don't forget, who did not really understand my hearing loss—because I'd never been honest with them.

Even in a more tempered situation, life for the spouse or partner of someone with hearing loss can be challenging. The British study found that partners played an important role in making the hearing-impaired person aware of the loss; that partners expected the hearing-impaired person to take some steps to help himself or herself, by wearing hearing aids, for instance; that they tried to protect their partner by ensuring that people who didn't know about the loss didn't perceive the behavior of the hearing-impaired person as rude.

The study also found that in couples where one person had

hearing loss both reported feelings of loneliness. Surprisingly, it was the hearing partner who felt most affected socially. "Hearing partners, in particular, spoke of feeling lonely and felt that they were missing out on companionship."

Spouses of the hard of hearing deserve a book of their own. Most of us who blog about our own experiences with hearing loss write about our spouses from time to time. Gael Hannan, whose blog "The Better Hearing Consumer"[62] is often hilariously right on target, refers to her spouse as the Hearing Husband. The Hearing Husband plays a role in many of her posts, and they even appeared together on a panel at the Canadian Hard of Hearing Association annual convention in 2014. Hannan's column is often laugh-out-loud funny, and also refreshingly honest.

Although this is not an actual conversation between the Hannans (or so Gael says), it is representative of the kind of "discussion"—i.e., argument—many of us have:

"Ex-CUSE me? I most certainly do not!"

"Why are you raising your voice... and what is it that you most certainly don't?"

"Oh, very funny... you know... what you just said... about what I do... because of my hearing loss!"

"What? All I said is sometimes you get things wrong, you don't hear them right, especially when you're upset... like now."

"Oh, like you don't? You implied that because I mis-hear some things, I make all conversations difficult."

"No, not all. But you have to admit that when you come out swinging at something you thought you heard, it can bung everything up."

"Do you think I like having this hearing loss? Don't you think that I'm trying my best, every minute of the day, to understand what's going on, to keep up? Do you know how draining that is? Do you?! And it doesn't help when, in the middle of a conversation, you turn away as you say something...."

"Why don't we calm down and..."

"Don't you tell me to calm down, you insensitive thug. You just don't care…."

Hannan goes on to offer some suggestions about minimizing the role of hearing loss in an argument: Face each other "eyeball to eyeball." If asked to repeat something, the hearing person should refrain from exaggerated enunciation, which will further inflame the hard-of-hearing (HOH) person. Argue only in well-lit spaces, where the HOH person is not at a disadvantage. Avoid yelling (see "further inflaming," above).

I am asked all the time about the best way to suggest to a spouse that he or she get a hearing checkup. This is a tough one. Try "Honey, I think you're having trouble with your hearing. You seem to be missing things." The response is invariably resistant: "No I'm not. My hearing is fine." Or "Maybe, but it doesn't bother me." Or "I hear fine. I just can't hear *you* because you mumble."

You could wait until the spouse brings the subject up. *Aha*, you think, when the spouse tentatively acknowledges a possible problem, *the opening I've been waiting for*. What you shouldn't do is leap in and say, "I've been telling you that for months!" and before the spouse has time to respond, pick up the phone to make an appointment with an audiologist.

"Lipreading Mom" (aka Shanna Groves) wrote a column about spousal hearing loss in 2013[63] in response to a reader who asked how to approach her husband about his hearing difficulties. She began by explaining a few things about people with hearing loss. "There is this other silent companion walking with a newly hard of hearing person. I call it MS. DENIAL. When we lose something dear to us, like our hearing, we often have the mentality, 'If I don't acknowledge it, then it doesn't exist.'" She went on to say that Ms. Denial is often soon joined by Mr. Anger, and shortly after by Miss Depression. "It could take your husband weeks, months or even longer to step away from MISS DEPRESSION's Icy Grip." But, finally, the day will come (or *may* come, in my opinion) when he says he thinks he might have hearing loss. "You nod," LipReading Mom advises. Do nothing for now. He's on his way to acceptance.

This would all be so much simpler if a hearing test were part of every annual physical. People are more willing to listen to a doctor than a spouse.

Tips for Caring for Kids When You Can't Hear Them

I already knew I had hearing loss when my husband and I decided to have children. My hearing loss was unilateral at the time, I didn't know it was progressive, and it never occurred to me that it might affect my ability to raise children. And it didn't. My two children, now twenty-eight and thirty-one, are fine, responsible, loving adults. Even if I'd known how serious the loss would get, I'd still have had children.

So it surprised me when I met a woman a few years ago who told me that she'd decided not to have children because of her hearing loss. It was especially surprising because we were in so many ways similar. We were the same age, our hearing loss and its progression was similar, we had the same audiologist, and we had both gotten hearing aids at the same time after a long delay. We lived in the same neighborhood, and she had even once lived in my building.

We both also had had fertility problems serious enough to prevent conceiving and carrying a child. My response, and my husband's, was to adopt. But Martha had taken her fertility problems as a sign that she wasn't meant to have children. She said she'd been worried she wouldn't be able to hear them.

That's understandable. In her 2014 memoir, *Not Fade Away*, Rebecca Alexander, who was going both blind and deaf from Usher Syndrome Type 3, addressed her concerns about having children. It's just about the only thing that seems to have given her pause. On top of having two master's degrees from Columbia and a thriving psychotherapy practice, she teaches spin classes and is, in general, upbeat, ambitious, and intrepid.

When it comes to having children, though, she hesitates. "I know how much a child can learn from having a parent who has a disability, and that it can instill a huge amount of compassion and empathy," she writes. But she worries the child would inevitably have to make compromises, would miss out on things, and would probably have to learn to do things independently before other children do. That's not what stops her: "[I would] never, ever want my children to feel the need to take care of me, or be my guide dog, or to ever feel like I couldn't take care of them."[64]

This is how Martha felt, I think. One of the most compelling books about living with hearing loss is Lou Ann Walker's *A Loss for Words*, about being the hearing child of profoundly deaf parents. Walker grew up in the fifties, and her parents were unsophisticated and relatively uneducated Midwesterners, though also deeply loving and a source of great support to their three hearing girls. There weren't many other deaf people around and her parents were misunderstood and belittled. Lou Ann acted as their interpreter from the time she learned to talk. It's a sad story, but it's also a story of a different period, long before Deaf Pride and Deaf Culture. Still, the description of young Lou Ann as her parents' guide dog is powerful and has probably imprinted itself on people with hearing loss even if they're not aware of it. But times have changed and—more important—so has technology.

Shanna Groves's "Lipreading Mom" blog is full of helpful advice, and she often answers readers' questions. As she wrote in one blog post:

"With my own family, I try to practice daily what I teach. My three school-age kids, who do not have hearing loss, make sure to face me and have my complete attention before talking to me. I remind them not to chat while chewing gum or food. Their mouths must always be in my line of sight when they want to have a conversation. A big

no-no is attempting to speech-read my kids through the rearview mirror while driving, or to speech-read when I am cooking at a hot stove or chopping food. Speech-reading requires full attention. As a mom with hearing loss, my communication motto is 'My eyes are my ears.'"

If I had young children now, with the severity of my hearing loss, I'd benefit from the technology that seems to have flooded the market in the past few years. Baby monitors come with flashing lights to show when the baby is crying. Some have a vibrating device that you can put under your pillow at night, belt clips so you can wear them when you're up, or even video so you can see the baby. Some let you talk to the baby, soothing him from afar without actually going into the room and waking him up. You can read more about these monitors on LiveStrong.com[65] and also on a website run by E-Michigan Deaf and Hard of Hearing People.[66] Many of these devices are useful to anyone with hearing loss whether they're a parent or not. I used a baby monitor when I stayed with my aged mother so that I could hear when she got out of bed.[67]

If you had hearing loss when your children were born, they've grown up with it and probably take it for granted. But if you lose your hearing in midlife, dealing with children can be more difficult. This is especially true if you're in denial about the loss. Middle- and high-school-age children find their parents inept and out of it in general, but if you're also saying "What?" all the time or misunderstanding them or if you're cranky and irritated about your hearing difficulties, relationships can fray pretty quickly. As in every situation, honesty helps. Be frank with your children about your hearing issues. You may be surprised by how graciously they rise to the occasion.

I met one of my favorite hard-of-hearing friends through our kids, both then in their early twenties. They were talking about their mothers and discovered that both had severe and recent hearing loss, so they put us together. We hit it off immediately.

I can find very little academic literature about the psycho-social impact of a parent or parents with hearing loss who are raising hearing children[68]—maybe because the situation has too many variables, including the age of onset of hearing loss relative to childrearing, whether one or both parents has hearing loss, the severity of the loss, etc. But because so much also depends on the personality of the parents, and on their attitude toward their hearing loss, it may be that no study could reliably assess the issues.

Being the Best Grandparent, No Matter Your Hearing Loss

'm not a grandparent yet, but I hope to be. I've always wanted to be a really involved grandparent, to have the grandkids come stay for weeks in the summertime while their parents work or take a vacation. I'd love to be one of those grandmothers who takes care of the grandkids once or twice a week. When they're older, I want to take them to Yosemite and Disney World.

Until I wrote this chapter, I thought those dreams would be unattainable for me. Why would any sane parent trust her young children with someone who couldn't hear them? But technology reassures me that I can do it. I just hope my kids think so, too.

Beyond confidence, there's another, more challenging, problem. Like many people with hearing loss, I have a very difficult time understanding young children. Baby talk is like a very strong foreign accent. Lisping makes it worse. Toddlers often talk very softy, except when they're screaming. I can't figure out the solution to that one.

I do hope that my grandchildren will come to understand that I'm a strong and competent grandmother, even though I can't hear everything. Five years ago, I was so demoralized by my hearing loss that I'd never have seen myself that way. It's been hard work shedding self-pity and self-loathing, and finding myself again, even if it's a self who has some limitations. Being honest and open and cheerful about my hearing loss was—and continues to be—essential. So is a sense of humor. Your grandchildren will appreciate it, too.

Caring for Elderly Dependent Parents

This is a situation I experienced when my hearing loss was at its very worst. In the time between when my hearing plunged, in 2008, and when I finally pulled myself together, in about 2012, my elderly parents both went through serious illnesses. I was their oldest child and the one who could travel most easily to where they lived, in South Carolina; those years are a blur of plane trips and ambulances and hospitals and nurse's aides hired and fired.

My father was diagnosed with lung cancer in 2008 and died in 2010. Until about six months before his death, he was my mother's sole caretaker. My mother graduated from Vassar (where she was a star onstage and in student government), raised four children practically on her own while my father traveled for his job and could do the Sunday *Times* crossword puzzle in an hour. But as she reached her eighties, she was beset with a host of health problems, including forgetfulness that developed into dementia; my father took it upon himself to care for her. He wouldn't have caregivers in the house, and as a consequence, either my mother or my father was always in a crisis or recovering from one.

I couldn't hear my mother, and even when I could catch her words, they might be garbled by her dementia. I could hear my father, who also had hearing loss (age-related in his case), but our conversations had to be loud for us to understand each other. My mother, with her perfect hearing, would hear us from a room away, discussing her health or, when my father's death became imminent, where she would live. She heard every word, and responded firmly that she wasn't going anywhere.

Health emergencies seemed to occur often: a fall, chest pain, a seizure. We'd call 911 and the house would be full of paramedics and firemen, their truck engines idling loudly in the driveway. In my panic (panic does not facilitate better hearing), I couldn't hear the paramedics over the trucks. Sometimes I thought I was the one they should take to the hospital. Audiologist Barbara Weinstein told me she has used a pocket talker to help paramedics communicate with people with hearing loss.

The worst was the night before my father died. I knew he was dying and had called to say I'd be arriving the next day. The hospice nurse handed him the phone and I said reassuring things, assuming he couldn't hear me and that he was unconscious. This was in the days before I had a captioned phone, and my hearing aid was pretty useless with the telephone. I hadn't expected him to say anything. Before I hung up, I said I'd see him tomorrow. "See you soon," he replied. Or at least I think he did. I'll never know for sure.

CHAPTER NINE

Dating:
Who, How, and When to Tell

"It's hard to feel romantic and attracted to someone who never seems to listen. But that's how someone with untreated hearing loss comes off."[69]
—*Sergei Kochkin*

I haven't dated for a good many years. And in fact I never really did date. I married my high school boyfriend and divorced him six years later, and then married my current husband with barely a date in between.

But I do know, from interviews and from meetings I've had with younger people with hearing loss, that dating poses special problems. This is also true for older people, of course—many of us are divorced or widowed or still single in our forties and fifties and sixties, and probably no more at ease on a first, second, or third date than we were in our twenties.

In February 2014, the website Cochlear Implant Online[70] published the results of a survey on "Dating, Relationships, Marriage

. . . and Hearing Loss." There were 192 respondents, 65 percent of whom described themselves as deaf and 35 percent as hard of hearing. (Interestingly, 21 percent of those with bilateral cochlear implants chose to identify themselves as "hard of hearing," though technically they were profoundly deaf in both ears.) Forty-nine percent of the respondents were married or in a domestic partnership. The survey didn't disclose age or specify which respondents answered which way, but it would be interesting to know if those who self-identified as "hard of hearing" had more positive dating/marriage experiences—and perhaps were more positive about life in general.

Almost all of the respondents (97 percent) used spoken language, but a quarter also used ASL or other sign language. The majority who were single didn't care whether they dated people with hearing loss (72 percent). The majority of married respondents were married to spouses with normal hearing and no family history of hearing loss (75 percent). It's important to remember that this was a cochlear implant website and probably included few if any respondents who identified as culturally Deaf, who would be more likely to want a culturally Deaf partner. But what we see from these respondents, who are functionally deaf or hard of hearing, is that the vast majority date and marry people who don't have hearing problems.

This may be partly logistical. If you live in a rural area or small town, you may not encounter others with hearing loss very often, especially not potential dates near your own age group. Even in a big city, because so many people aren't open about their loss, you may have a hard time knowing who has hearing loss and who doesn't.

One way to meet others with hearing loss is to go to meetings of groups like HLAA or ALDA. If your area has a local or state chapter of HLAA, sign up to join the annual Walk4Hearing, a fun event and a great way to meet others with hearing loss. Another way might be to join support groups run by the military, because hearing loss and tinnitus are an enormous problem for veterans.

I'm married to a hearing person, and I can say with some authority that there are pluses and minuses. The minuses first, because they really are pretty minor: My husband will never truly understand what my hearing loss is like, despite decades of marriage and a great deal of writing about it on my part. But maybe someone with hearing loss wouldn't, either: We all hear differently, depending on the nature and severity of our loss, how well we respond to hearing aids and cochlear implants, and what we expect from our hearing.

The pluses easily override the minuses. I like having someone around who can hear at night, when I have my hearing aid and implant out. I especially like this when we are in our isolated house in the country. If I didn't have a hearing spouse, I'd get around this in other ways: I'd install an alarm system with flashing lights. I'd have my doorbell and phone and anything else wired to flash rather than ring or buzz. I bet I could even set my kitchen timer to respond visually. I might have houseguests more often. I'd also have a trained service dog.

Instead, my dog is primarily a pet (though he does have a helpfully loud bark). I do have a captioned telephone and a fire alarm that shakes the bed (often when I simply burn food in the kitchen). Still, I feel better with a hearing spouse around. In addition, as one of the respondents in the Cochlear Implant Online survey said, "It makes my life easier. I know that may sound selfish, but I depend on my guy to hear the things I cannot when we go out in public."

When to Tell

Because most people don't meet dates through hearing loss groups, there may be no indication that they have hearing loss. Hearing loss, as we know, is an invisible condition—up to a point. This is an important issue in many social and professional situations, including job interviews, and it's never an easy one. More than half the respondents in the Cochlear Implant Online survey (53 percent) said they told dates about their hearing loss before the first date, and another 30 percent did so on the second date. If you have a cochlear implant, you don't usually have a choice about whether or when to disclose. Cochlear implants tend to be visible. So this may skew the results on this survey a bit.

Another thing that may influence the relatively large number of people who tell either before or on the first date is the presumed age group of the respondents. Young people who have grown up with hearing loss tend to be more comfortable with it. It's harder for a forty-five-year-old who has been hearing all her life and suddenly has severe hearing loss to be as open about it.

If you're a passionate and outspoken advocate for hearing awareness, it's a no-brainer. Others are more cautious, wanting a date to get to know them "as a person" before raising the issue of hearing loss. For instance, if you meet someone through a dating website, it's probably better to wait for an in-person meeting to bring up the subject.

Hearing loss also affects the kind of dates you go on. Most people with serious hearing loss have trouble hearing at big parties or at bars. More than half of the respondents said it was a consideration when choosing places to go for dates. All in all, these respondents seemed upbeat about the experience. One noted that her hearing loss had brought her closer to partners who were "willing to work with my extra needs and start to form their habits to help my hearing loss." Another cautioned: "Hearing aids make great jerk screeners," adding, "if he can't see you past the hearing aids, he's not a good catch."

The decision about when and what to tell is ultimately about honesty in the relationship. If you can't be honest about your hearing loss with a particular individual, the relationship will suffer.

Dating While in Denial

Because the majority of people with hearing loss in the United States are under the age of sixty, with most of them having begun to lose their hearing between twenty and fifty-nine, it's not that surprising that many of them find it difficult to be open about their hearing loss. And because only one person in seven who could benefit from hearing aids has one, many HOH people don't have that particular clue to give them away.

Sergei Kochkin, formerly the executive director of the Better Hearing Institute and a strong advocate for people with hearing loss, wrote a column on sex with hearing loss, which I quoted at the beginning of this chapter. "You've devoted time and attention to improving your sex life. But you are probably ignoring a small electronic device that could really light a fire in your intimate relationships." No, it's not what you're thinking. "It's a hearing aid."

Kochkin goes on to note that most couples' therapists put effective communication at the top of a "must" list for a good relationship. This is true not only in committed relationships but for new ones as well.

Although you may want to wait till the potential new partner gets to know you as a person before you tell him or her about your hearing loss, remember that you may never get to that point if you come off as bored or uninterested. Or, if you're older, if he or she thinks you might be going gaga.

Being open about hearing loss also helps in planning dates. If your date still wants to go to a noisy restaurant or a big party every time you go out, even after you've told him about your hearing loss, he's probably not right for you.

One other piece of advice: Bluffing can have disastrous consequences. As one hearing aid site wrote: "Did he just say 'I love you' or 'I love juice'?" Taking a wild guess could make you look ridiculous and might even end something promising.

What to Watch Out For

Some hearing people actively seek out deaf or hard of hearing people to date. Their motivations are varied. Some may simply find deafness weird and fascinating. "That makes me feel like a carnival attraction," wrote one woman in a chat group on AllDeaf.com. Others may want to date you because it makes them look heroic: The deaf partner is a kind of status symbol.

It gets uglier: "I find that most hearing men who are attracted to us Deaf women think we are easy to 'control,'" wrote one woman on AllDeaf.com. "One time a guy with shit for brains told me: 'I was really glad when I found out you were deaf. When I saw Marlee Matlin for the first time, I thought to myself, 'Wouldn't it be great to have a Deaf woman. I bet they don't talk or nag as much as hearing women.'" Not only is that offensive and stupid, it's also wrong: Deaf women talk and nag as much as anyone. And so do Deaf men.

Not surprisingly, people with hearing loss may attract those who are downright nuts. Yes, deaf wannabees do exist (just as do people who want to be amputees). They even have a group in the U.K., called Deaf Wannabees. A discussion on the website Grumpy Old Deafies yielded some surprisingly thoughtful comments. Should health-care resources be allocated to people who pretend to be deaf or who actually manage to deafen themselves? One comment was especially provocative: "If we [people who are deaf or hard of hearing] say we're human beings of value, then why do so many condemn someone who wants to be deaf? Are we really saying that deep down deafness is never okay, and therefore no one should have a desire to become deaf?"

And, finally, hearing aid fetishists: In a 2007 study, researchers at the University of Bologna[71] did a large-scale study on fetishes, based on a complicated formula involving participants in Internet chat groups. Foot and shoe fetishes were the most common (47 percent preferred feet and 32 percent preferred shoes). But hearing aids garnered more perverse interest than you might expect: 150 of those surveyed (less than 1 percent) expressed a penchant for hearing aids. Either to wear them, hold them, smell them, or even have them fitted. This was less than a quarter of the number with diaper fetishes, but much bigger than the number of those with a fetish for catheters or pacemakers.

Sex While Wearing Hearing Aids

Do you keep them in? There's always the risk of shrieks and squeals, but that's true even with an old friend who greets you with a big kiss on both cheeks. You might worry about a hearing aid coming loose and falling out. Sweat isn't good for hearing aids.

In general, the answer seems to be "take them out."

If you take them out, how do you communicate—especially in the dark? There are ways, as we all know.

Needless to say, it's probably a good idea before you get to this point to disclose your hearing loss and talk about communication.

· CHAPTER TEN ·

You Gotta Have Friends

But you may have to work harder to keep them.

Hearing loss can take a toll on friendships. It can become difficult to maintain the kind of relationship you've had with even your close friends as your hearing deteriorates. The kinds of activities you shared may not work for you anymore. But it's important not to isolate yourself. You have to find new ways to interact with old friends. And you may also have to find some new friends. Luckily, hearing loss itself offers opportunities to meet new people. The most obvious is by joining a support group. Both HLAA and ALDA have local chapters across the country. The meetings will have hearing assistance, usually in the form of live captioning projected onto a screen at the front of the room, a technology known as Caption Access Real-Time, or Communication Access Real-Time (CART). Some of the meeting spaces are also looped. If a chapter has Deaf members, there will be an ASL interpreter.

The first time I went to a chapter meeting of HLAA, I looked around at the group and almost backed out. They all looked so old! Even the young ones looked old. But I quickly realized that that was just the stigma of age distorting my vision. I expected to see old and that's what I saw.

In fact the New York City chapter of HLAA is made up of adults of all ages, with a strong contingent in their very energetic fifties and sixties, and other members as young as their twenties. As I've become more active in the group, joining in advocacy activities, going to captioned theater and musical performances, becoming a board member, I've come to count quite a few of my HLAA acquaintances as friends, real friends.

Some hear better than I do, some hear worse. Some use extra devices in addition to hearing aids or cochlear implants to facilitate their hearing. Some can't hear at all and read lips. (Most of us don't know sign language.) Almost all of us use smartphone apps to resort to written notes if we can't make ourselves understood. Some use Dragon Dictation. Others use Siri. Some use other apps, and some even use plain old pencil and paper. Sometimes communication is frustrating, but we can usually laugh about it.

Recently, I was asked to give a talk at a benefit for a law firm that does a lot of pro bono work for the deaf and hard of hearing. The benefit was held in a Chelsea art gallery, all cement walls and floors. Acoustic hell. I didn't recognize many of the people when I walked in, and I couldn't hear anything anyone said to me. But then my hearing loss friends started showing up. They came partly to support the law firm but also to support me. Many of them had been at an earlier gathering that day at another organization honoring one of our members for her volunteer work. I'm very happy to have these new friends.

True Friendship Survives Hearing Loss

My close friends always knew about my hearing loss. None of them knew the extent of it, though they did sometimes feel the brunt of it.

As my hearing loss worsened in my late fifties and early sixties, and my mood darkened, I was not an easy person to be around. I was irrationally angry at my hearing friends for not being careful enough about how they talked to me, even though I'd never told them what I needed. One friend insisted on leaning into my ear and talking, which obviously makes speech reading impossible. She did it more than once in the middle of a performance in a darkened theater. It drove me crazy. Instead of being open and forthright—and specific—I'd simply hiss at her, "I can't hear you!"

My hearing friends, I'm sure, often thought I wasn't listening, or not paying attention. They might even have thought I just didn't care about the friendship.

For my part, I relied more and more on email to communicate, and I was hurt or miffed when the friend never got around to emailing back.

Realizing that I was responsible for these rifts, these hurt feelings, was a big part of my recovery from hearing loss. I was the one who had let the friendships lapse. It was my responsibility to renew them.

At first, I saw my friends mostly one on one, instead of at the group lunches or book club meetings or dinner parties where most of our socializing had previously taken place.

One on one, I could hear in a way I couldn't in a group. But beyond that, conversation between two people is inevitably more intimate. I told them more about my hearing loss, and I explained what worked for me and what didn't. The friend who always whispered in my ear started carrying a little notepad to fill me in on words I'd missed in a conversation.

I rejoined my book club, and one friend, who declared herself the "conversation bitch," made sure we talked one at a time so I could hear—and also kept us on the subject: the book.

Not surprisingly, these old friendships not only revived but deepened. As I began to confide my own problems, my friends became more open about theirs. My friendships became intimate and mutually supportive. We were able to talk about personal things in a meaningful way, but also about issues and ideas, something that is always hard for me in a group.

I still can't hear confidences (often whispered), can't pick up jokes, miss whole chunks of conversation, and occasionally I simply decline to show up in the first place. But my friendships are truer and stronger than they ever were before.

Most of them.

The stress inflicted on a friendship by hearing loss can reveal underlying flaws in the relationship. A few years ago, a friend told me that she didn't want to keep up our regular walk routine in part because I couldn't hear her. (The other part was because of my dog, an occasionally boisterous companion.) That was painful. We had always had stimulating, thought-provoking conversations on our long walks—sometimes gossip, sometimes about our families and friends, sometimes about work conflicts and strategies to deal with them, and sometimes debates about politics and policy and philosophy and books. I felt I heard most of it. But what she said made me realize how vexed our relationship already was, hearing loss aside. The friendship was taking too much emotional energy and resulting in too many hard feelings. We both let it taper off.

My drop into severe hearing loss coincided with several family crises, and with work crises as well. Each was difficult in itself, but combined they led to depression and social isolation on the one hand, and frenetic activity and anxiety dealing with family and work on the other. I didn't have time for friends. I didn't let them help me.

Eventually, the family crises were resolved, mostly—alas—

through the death over three years of five close family members, all of whom had been chronically ill. My work crises ended with my leaving my job. I began seeing a therapist who treated my depression and anxiety and, perhaps most important, encouraged me to come out about my hearing loss.

And I found my friends again.

Good Friends Make for Better Health

Untreated hearing loss has well-documented social-psychological effects. One of these is social isolation. The National Institute on Aging has found a significantly greater incidence of social isolation and depression in those with hearing loss. Social isolation and situational depression can be treated by, first, correcting the hearing loss. Depression that results from hearing loss can be treated with short-term therapy that helps you understand the grieving process, understand that grieving is normal, and know that acceptance of the loss is possible.

Once you address these two admittedly major issues, social isolation usually corrects itself. Sometimes you need to give yourself a push. Social isolation becomes habit-forming. It's important to break that habit.

Friendships and social connections are a key factor in living a longer healthy life. This was demonstrated in "The Longevity Project," a book-length report on an eighty-year study of 1,528 individuals that began with Dr. Lewis Terman in 1921 and was completed by Drs. Howard S. Friedman and Leslie Martin. In a 2011 interview, I asked Dr. Friedman and Dr. Martin what the single strongest social predictor of long life was. Their unhesitating answer: a strong social network.[72]

People with hearing loss sometimes have to make themselves keep up those social connections. If you know you're not going to be able to hear at a lecture, a party, or a restaurant, the tendency is to stay home. This is true also of places of worship. It's one reason why looping, which I'll discuss in Chapter 20, is so important. (For a quick definition, see the Glossary.)

Lectures, classes, and worship services are places where many of us go for social, intellectual, and spiritual stimulation. It's where we meet new people, and hear new ideas. If a venue like a lecture hall or place of worship is looped, it becomes accessible to those with hearing loss simply by a flip of the T-coil switch on their hearing aid.

These are also the kind of places where friendships are formed and nurtured. We need to be sure they are accessible to those with hearing loss. Your local chapter of the Hearing Loss Association of America may have a list of looped venues.[73] A looped venue is a good place to start getting yourself out and about again.

Join a Like-Minded Group

As I said at the beginning of this chapter, hearing loss offers opportunities for friendship: Your local chapter of HLAA or ALDA, or any kind of support group that deals with hearing loss, is a good place to start making friends. A list of these chapters is available on the HLAA website[74] and the ALDA website.[75]

The first time I went to a chapter meeting of HLAA, I hung back and didn't really talk to anybody. There was a guest speaker, and thanks to the CART screen and the hearing loop, I could follow even from the back of the room, where I'd skulked, hoping to go unnoticed. I wasn't ready at that point to declare myself a person with hearing loss. But it really took just that one meeting to encourage me to come back.

HLAA chapter meetings often have guest speakers. Our New York City chapter has regular panel discussions. The topics range from hearing aids and assistive technology (these panels are made up of audiologists and other experts) to theater access (the panel included a representative from the Theatre Development Fund, which provides live captioning in Broadway and off-Broadway theaters, and several theater-access advocates). We've had meetings to discuss progress in other advocacy initiatives, for instance the effort to get movie theaters looped. I myself have been the invited speaker at chapter meetings around the country.

One of the best parts of these meetings is that everyone wears a name tag. Another pleasure is to be able to hear, via looping (or reading on the CART screen), everything that is said. It's hard for hearing people to understand how frustrating it is to attend an event where you can't hear the speaker. How many commencement addresses and panel discussions and award citations have I sat through without understanding a single word?

To go to an event where I can "hear"—that's rare.

I also didn't realize at first how valuable I would find meeting people who were confronting many of the same issues I was. Who understood why I was having trouble. Who shared tips and hints about getting along more easily in a hearing world.

This chapter of the book is about friendship, though, not advocacy. So what is HLAA doing here? It's because through HLAA I have a whole new group of friends. They are all members of the New York City chapter, and I'd probably have met none of them if I hadn't started going to the monthly chapter meetings. These are people I think of as real friends, not simply hearing loss acquaintances. There are dozens of those, too.

How many people can make dozens of new friends and acquaintances in their mid-sixties? It's hard enough for anyone, and even harder for people with hearing loss—at least until you acknowledge it. And then everything changes. Before, I was losing friends because of my hearing loss, but now, I'm gaining them.

CHAPTER ELEVEN

The Job Search

Get your foot in the door before you mention hearing loss.

Almost all experts recommend that you not disclose your hearing loss on a résumé. People have preconceptions and prejudices about hearing loss. There's a good chance you won't get past the résumé stage unless, of course, it's a job related to hearing loss. Then it's a plus.

That's the only hard and fast rule. Like most everything else having to do with hearing loss, many factors affect looking for a job.

If you have mild to moderate hearing loss, the first step should be to get a hearing aid. Most hearing aids these days are virtually invisible, and for people with mild to moderate hearing loss they can fully restore hearing. If your hearing is perfect with a hearing aid, there is no reason whatsoever to disclose the hearing loss. Unless it affects job performance, it's nobody's business.

Sometimes a hearing test is included in a pre-employment physical. Unless the hearing loss will affect your ability to carry out the essential functions of the job, a discovery of hearing loss is irrelevant. The fact that you haven't mentioned it is also irrelevant. At this point, because you have already been offered the job before you took the physical, you are protected by the Americans with Disabilities Act. Nevertheless, *essential* is a subjective term. See the end of this chapter for more on this.

If your hearing loss is more severe, then you're faced with the difficult decision about when to disclose, how much to say about it, and at what point to ask for accommodations.

Don't Trip Yourself Up in the Résumé

CBS News MoneyWatch's Suzanne Lucas offers a list of "Don'ts" in writing a résumé. One of them is "Don't share too much information. No birthdate, religion, hobbies, weight, social security number, marital status, links to Facebook or personal blog, children, sexual orientation, or life mission statements."[76] To that I would include no information about hearing loss.

You do need to research the job you're applying for and make sure that the primary responsibilities are things you can do. If your hearing loss is serious, you probably shouldn't apply for a job in a busy call center where there will be lots of overlapping voices. If you're intent on that job, however, and think you'd be good at it despite the loss, go ahead and apply—but in the interview you should discuss the fact that you may need a captioned phone.

Other jobs are probably off limits to someone with poor hearing. You wouldn't make a good court stenographer. If your hearing loss is significant, you probably want to skip applying for work as an airline pilot. But even these are jobs you may be able to hold on to if you develop hearing loss after you're employed. You may be able to adopt strategies to cope with the loss.

If you decide not to disclose your hearing loss on your résumé, make sure that you're not then disclosing it inadvertently. A young woman named Sarah Honigfeld wrote a column on the Boston Chapter of HLAA's website about her experience applying and interviewing for a job.[77] Generally open about her hearing loss, she had decided not to disclose it on her résumé but to wait for an opportunity to discuss it in person at an interview. A Deaf friend pointed out several telltale references on her résumé that were a tip-off to her deafness: She noted that she was fluent in ASL, that she had worked as a classroom aid for Deaf children, that she'd worked at a nonprofit with Deaf college students. She could perfectly well be interested in working with the Deaf without being Deaf herself, but it may have kept her from getting past the résumé stage. "Realizing this made me rethink some of my job applications and how my résumé may have impacted my chances of being asked to interview for a job," she said later.

Honigfeld went on to discuss a situation where she had been called in for an individual interview, which went well, and then for a second, group interview. At this point, she requested a sign-language interpreter, which she paid for. "During the interview, it was obvious how awkward and uneasy everyone felt with the interpreter, and I ended up bombing the interview. As expected, I wasn't offered the job."

As it turned out, the group was smaller than she'd anticipated and she probably could have managed by reading lips. But she didn't regret the decision to bring in the interpreter: "If this company couldn't get over having a person in the room signing... then I wasn't interested in spending a year of my time there." Although willing to help raise awareness in the workplace, she wrote, "I didn't feel like forcing the issue with employers that didn't want to accept me in the first place."

Erin Geld was born deaf in one ear and nearly deaf in the other, had been mainstreamed in school, and was up-front about disclosing her hearing loss and asking for help when she needed it. But, as she wrote in an article on Monster.com,[78] when it came to writing a résumé, she decided not to disclose her hearing loss. "I am extremely capable in terms of communication and language—I use the phone, am a serious chatterbox, and love to write." Even though Geld sees her hearing loss as an important part of her personality that "indicates a certain strength, patience, humility, and perseverance," she decided to omit the information, knowing that not everyone sees hearing loss in the positive light she does.

She worried that a more negative stereotype might come to mind: "mumbling, awkwardly squawking half-wit." But her hearing loss and nondisclosure tripped her up when the employer, "a very cool consulting company," set up a phone interview. The questions were tough: "Give me a two-minute pitch on your favorite consumer gadget." "What do you think are the chances of Microsoft buying out Yahoo?" Afterward, she realized she should have told the interviewer from the start that she had a hearing loss and suggested other interview methods: an online chat, an in-person interview.

After that experience, she rewrote her résumé, adding a section titled "Background and Languages," which included the fact that she had dual Brazilian-American citizenship and a British education, was bilingual, and also, last, was "hearing disabled." In addition, she had a good GPA and a strong leadership background. She didn't get many responses, but she attributed that in part to a very competitive job market in San Francisco.

Eventually, she applied for a job in education, which included an essay. She took the opportunity to write frankly about her hearing loss, including the fact that her own experience would be a benefit in a classroom. "I argued that I would have a special understanding of the learning child, as I am constantly learning myself." She got the job.

The Interview: Prepare for the Unexpected

J oyce Bender, who owns a search firm in Pittsburgh that places many people with disabilities, advises avoiding disclosure in the interview as well, if possible. As Sarah Honigfeld's experience shows, it's not always possible.

My advice to a job applicant would be to come to the interview prepared to disclose, and to think in advance how that disclosure might benefit you. You may find yourself seated for the interview next to a humming fish tank or a noisy air conditioner (both have happened to me). Casually suggest moving your chair, with a vague reference to the fish tank muffling the interviewer's voice. If you are seated so that the interviewer is framed by bright light, making it impossible to speech-read, say the light is in your eyes and you'd like to move. This is true, if only part of the truth.

What if you find yourself in an interview with one of those impossible to understand people (mustache, mumbler, thin lips)? At that point, it's probably better to acknowledge a degree of hearing loss and pull out your FM system—a device that will transmit the interviewer's voice to your hearing aid or cochlear implant—or one of the new microphone/transmitters like Phonak's Roger (both are discussed in Chapter 18). Simply put it on the desk and explain what it is. Then ignore the device as you accurately hear and answer the interviewer's questions. You may want to assure him or her that it's not a tape recorder.

A prospective employer suggests lunch in a restaurant or over a drink. Say you're sensitive to noise and you'd rather meet where you'll be able to hear him easily. This won't work if the job itself involves a lot of work lunches and schmoozing over drinks—at that point hearing in a noisy bar can be considered an essential component of the job.

Telephone interviews are increasingly common. If you don't want to acknowledge the hearing loss and can't avoid the phone interview, make sure you take the call on a captioned phone.

As for group interviews, I wince even to think of them. Practice in advance. Get a group of friends together, put your FM transmitter on the table, set it to pick up surrounding noise, encourage your friends to talk normally, even occasionally interrupting one another, and see how you do. Then if you find yourself in a difficult situation during the real interview, say, sitting around a table with six eager interviewers, you'll be prepared. Take out your FM transmitter, explain what it is, briefly and efficiently, and then hope everyone forgets it's there on the table. Again, if big meetings are an essential component of the job, and if the FM system doesn't help all that much, the employer has a legitimate reason to turn you down.

Valerie Stafford-Mallis, who lost her hearing after she was in the workforce and now wears two cochlear implants, says her personal advice is always to be honest up front. "My experience was people were more accepting of the hearing loss when I simply presented it as one of many aspects of my uniqueness. I found that when I mentioned it *after* I struggled with the communication, it called more attention to the fact that I struggled." Stafford-Mallis, who serves on the HLAA board with me, works with the business community in Florida and elsewhere on issues surrounding the deaf and hard of hearing, so her advice makes perfect sense for her situation. Others, working in non-hearing-related fields, might feel that holding back on this information is the wiser strategy, at least for the short term.

ADA Protection Has Limits

Employers don't need legitimate reasons to turn you down. They don't have to give reasons at all. Even if you disclose your hearing loss, ask for an ASL interpreter or CART services for the interview, or put your FM system on the table, they still don't have to offer you the job. The Americans with Disabilities Act, as the Hearing Loss Association of America's excellent Employment Toolkit[79] points out, "is not an affirmative action law; it does not require the establishment of hiring or promotion goals for people with disabilities."

Once you are offered the job, the employer can ask medical questions and can require a medical examination. But it can't be targeted just to you. The medical exam has to be required for all new hires applying for the same kind of position. The medical exam may include a hearing test if the employer deems a particular level of hearing proficiency essential to the job, and if the hearing test is given to all new hires in this area.

You can wear hearing aids during the test, although an employer may claim that wearing hearing aids while on the job poses a risk to yourself or others. This was the issue in the NYPD case that I mentioned earlier. New York City settled after the plaintiffs made an airtight case for allowing police officers to take the mandatory hearing test with their hearing aids. If they could pass the test, their ability to perform the job would be considered on a case-by-case basis.[80]

The other legitimate reason to turn you down at this point is if the employer can prove that because of your hearing loss you are unable to perform the "essential functions" of the job even with reasonable accommodations. The employer can withdraw the offer. Although the ADA (and the Rehabilitation Act for federal employees) prohibits discrimination against qualified employees with disabilities, the term "qualified" is open to interpretation. As the HLAA toolkit says, "Only apply for jobs for which you are qualified."

CHAPTER TWELVE

Once You Get the Job

Congratulations! Now comes the hard part.

The first weeks in a new job, or even in a new position with the same employer, are always difficult. You probably have a whole new set of coworkers whose personalities and status you need to sort out over the next few days or weeks. You may be using a new computer system. The daily schedules and routines are unfamiliar.

Most people will be helpful, especially if you ask. But there's always the office grouch who will assume that you've already been told that Item X goes into Slot Y, with a cover letter, copied and filed. The next day you'll be faced with Item M. Didn't Office Grouch mention that, too, when she was chewing you out about Item X? Ask again (though don't ask Ms. Grouch): Item M goes into Box Q, no cover letter. It will be copied and filed at the end of the week by a clerk whose job it is to keep Box Q up-to-date. If you copy and file yourself, you'll mess up the clerk's system.

Even ordinary routines have to be relearned: Where does your coat go, and is part of the closet reserved for some special people? What do people wear? Are sandals acceptable? Do women show their toes? Do the men wear sneakers or do you have to find some dress shoes? Is it okay to eat at your desk? What's acceptable in terms of personal phone calls? How often can you take a bathroom break before it gets noticeable? How tidy does your desk need to be? Where are the mailboxes and when are deliveries? Who opens the mail—especially if a lot of packages arrive daily? How do you mail a letter? Where are the recycling bins? Do people take smoke breaks, and if so where do they go? Do you have to get to work early or is it okay to show up on time? If you're a few minutes late, how big a transgression is that? What's the usual lunch break—when and for how long? Do people work beyond the official end of the day? Is that expected?

Getting accustomed to the culture of an office, or a new department, is stressful. It's even more stressful if you hear poorly.

Where to Sit

The location of your desk or cubicle can make all the difference in how well you do in terms of hearing. Assuming you've decided not to be up-front about your hearing loss, you need to figure out how you can best function in this particular office environment, including finding a relatively quiet place to work.

If you can, try to make these arrangements before your first day on the job. Once you're assigned a desk or cubicle, it's harder to change it.

This takes some creative observing and thinking. If the interview has taken place in the office, try to take notice of the surroundings before you leave. Note areas that would be especially difficult for you. Is the copy machine or the fax machine in the middle of the room? You want to be as far away as possible. Is there a central hub where meetings and informal gatherings take place? You might want to be at a distance so the noise doesn't bother you, or you might want to be as close as possible so you always know what's going on. Are there heavily trafficked areas or places where people congregate and chatter?

How do you express these preferences without acknowledging your hearing loss? In my opinion, this is where you take the first step toward what might eventually be full disclosure. It's good to lay the groundwork.

When you meet your new manager on the first day, say how much you're looking forward to the job and how [choose your adjective: inviting, beautiful, excitingly busy] the workspace is. If you spot a problem when she shows you your desk, this is the time to mention that you sometimes have trouble hearing in noise and might it be possible to work farther away from the elevator/copier/telephone bank/coffee machine/water cooler?

If the response is that that's the only space available, say you understand and ask the manager casually if she can keep the request in mind in case a new desk opens up. I think of this kind of comment as a putting a small wedge into a door you may want to push open wider later on. The manager probably won't remember why you wanted a different desk (and probably not even the fact that you asked for a different desk), but in the back of her mind is a vague awareness of something about hearing. I love the phrase "the camel's nose under the tent." Usually, it's used as a warning that once the camel gets its nose under, before long it'll be in your sleeping bag with you. But you can see it from the camel's perspective. You're the camel. Your comment is the nose under the tent.

Unwelcome Surprises

Once you've figured out the customs and routines of the office, you may realize that the job poses more hearing obstacles than you expected. Maybe there's more telephone work than you thought there would be. Maybe you are expected to travel and communicate by cell phone. Maybe office work often spills over to the neighborhood bar after work. Maybe office-wide gatherings of a hundred or more people take place more often than you thought they would, and you have a hard time hearing the speaker. Maybe the person in the next cubicle has a booming voice, which he uses all day long.

The best solution to this kind of problem is to acknowledge your hearing loss and ask for accommodations. Indeed, if you want to be protected by the Americans with Disabilities Act, you must do that. But disclosure is double-edged: It can assure you protections under the ADA and probably get you accommodations. But you also run the risk of being seen as someone with a disability—before you've had a chance to prove yourself on the job. Many people choose to establish themselves first as competent and efficient workers— maybe even invaluable workers!—before they disclose their hearing loss.

There are some ways to get past these obstacles without disclosing—at least not disclosing before your trial period is up.

The Telephone

Ah, my nemesis.

Does your hearing aid have a T-coil? If not, get one. Is your office telephone T-coil compatible? It has to be, by law, but the electromagnetic signal put out by the phone may not be strong enough to transmit the sound clearly to your hearing aid. In this case, you may have to ask for a different phone (which means a degree of disclosure).

If the telecoil is strong enough, your telephone problems are resolved. Before you answer or make a call, you flip the switch on your hearing aid to the telecoil program. If you don't have a switch on the hearing aid, you can do this using a remote. You can also use a neckloop with a telecoil, but that's going to be a tip-off if you don't want to disclose yet.

The telecoil turns off the hearing aid microphone so it excludes most other noise in the room. The speaker's voice goes directly to the hearing aid. The downside of this is that if you forget to switch the T-coil off after the call, you won't be able to hear the next person who speaks to you. Some hearing aids include what's called an "MT" setting, which allows simultaneous access to signals picked up by the T-coil and the microphone. When your hearing aid is set on the MT option, you can hear room sounds while on the telephone.

Phone headsets can also be T-coil compatible. Many office workers use headsets, which helps if you do not wish to disclose your hearing loss, but there's still the concern that the signal from the phone may not be strong enough. I found, as a nondiscloser, that the headset itself was much more effective than the handheld phone. (My hearing aid at that point did not have a telecoil.) It was also much easier on my neck—no cricks from balancing a phone receiver on your shoulder all day. Still, as you will see in Chapter 13, this was not a sustainable solution for me. I should have fessed up and asked for a captioned phone.

Cell Phones

Whether you're traveling, running late, or making a call from home, you'll have to use a cell phone at some point. Don't assume the phone is hearing aid compatible. Hearing aid compatible (HAC) means that it is wired to work with your hearing aid and telecoil. In the regular microphone mode, the wiring should prevent static or buzzing. In telecoil mode, the signal should be clear.

Most iPhones were not HAC until the iPhone 5 came along. (See Chapter 18 for more specific information on hearing aid compatibility.) In general, if you're looking for a hearing aid–compatible phone, look for one with a ranking of at least M3/T3 (for microphone and telecoil). These will be on the label next to the sample phone in the store, which tells you its features.

People with hearing loss probably also want to be sure the phone can receive texts and email—and should know how to use them. Captioning is another option. A new system called Innocaptions, or InnoCapTalk, was surprisingly accurate and efficient in translating voice to captions. The main drawback was that the caller had to use a special assigned telephone number, a bother if you'd had the same cell phone number for years. Also, on some brands of smartphone, and with some carriers, you couldn't get voice plus captioning unless you also had Wi-Fi. Most people use cell phones when there isn't Wi-Fi—on the street, for instance. So you had to choose between voice and captions. As of mid-May 2015, Innocaptions suspended service "until further notice," and its CEO, Chuck Owen, sent an emotional letter to all subscribers announcing his departure.

Meetings

Everybody hates meetings, but the person who can't hear hates them the most. Assuming that most of the meetings you attend take place in a conference room, you can do several things to maximize your ability to understand what's being discussed.

Try to sit with your back to the window or any bright source of light. If the person speaking is across the table from you and backlit, you'll never be able to read his lips. If it's a rectangular or oval table with the speaker at the head, try to put yourself about halfway down the longer side. If one ear is better than the other, try to have that ear facing the direction of the principal speaker.

Sometimes you can't do all of these at once. If sitting with your right ear closer to the principal speaker means facing the window with five other people's faces backlit, you have to weigh the options: Maybe the boss or the person who is leading the meeting has an especially clear voice—whew, problem solved. Maybe he or she has a quiet voice, an accent, a mustache, etc. In that case, sit as close to the speaker as possible.

Unfortunately, though, there is no easy solution to this. How to manage in meetings is one of the questions I'm most frequently asked.

It's always helpful to ask for an agenda for the meeting and, if anyone is taking notes, ask to see the notes afterward. When I was leading meetings, I'd always ask someone else to take notes and distribute them to everyone (including me, most important!).

Even if you have disclosed your loss, solutions aren't easy. My audiologist was always urging me to get a receiver that would pick up the speech from all meeting participants, as long as they wore a small microphone I'd provided. This is fine if you're the CEO. Much harder to ask everyone to wear a lapel mic if you're in the vast middle of the ranks.

You can try putting the transmitter from your FM system, set to pick up sound from every direction, discreetly on the table. If the room is small enough and the acoustics are good, and if people speak clearly enough and one at a time, this might be adequate. If you have Phonak's new Roger system, which I discuss in Chapter 18, you'll have even more of an advantage.

Meetings are one area where disclosure can be very helpful. If your attendance at the meetings is not essential, explain the issue to your supervisor and ask if you can simply have someone brief you afterward. If your presence is essential, ask for CART. Your boss may balk at this but you can mention some of the benefits of CART—not only to you but to the company as well: A CART transcript is saved on the operator's computer and can be used later as minutes of the meeting, or as raw material for writing up the minutes. CART transcripts are confidential and cannot be distributed to anyone not authorized to receive them. They can be destroyed after the meeting if the supervisor wishes it.

The cost of CART services varies, in most areas $125 to $150 an hour, even in expensive cities like New York. That may seem like a lot in a small company, but unless the company can come up with another solution or show that the cost is prohibitive, it's a violation of the ADA to require the employee to attend the meeting without CART support.

Large meetings in a conference center or hotel ballroom require different strategies. One tech-savvy friend, who asked that his name not be used, told me he always begins by getting to the session early and talking with the audiovisual technicians. He plugs his FM transmitter into the AV board out jack. The sound then goes directly from the AV board via his FM system to a receiver connected to his cochlear implant. It would work similarly with hearing aids. Phonak's Roger, which works on a GHz system,[81] is even easier to use. Cochlear is also about to introduce a 2.4 GHz transmitter. For meetings at a large conference table, my friend says he may use two or more Roger pens, which I will explain further in Chapter 18. On a lower-tech level, he makes sure that conference participants all wear name tags with their names on the front and on the back, if they're on lanyards.

How about teleconferencing? If the speakers are using Skype, you have the advantage of being able to watch their lips. Skype also has a good audio system, as do other Internet based phone services like GoToMeeting. If it's purely an audio conference . . . well, I have no suggestions for that one except to somehow figure out if you can call in from your home phone and then make sure it's a captioned one.

Bluffing requires not only stamina but also creativity.

Happy Hour

This is a big problem not only for those with hearing loss but for many others with hidden disabilities. A recovering alcoholic may not want to be around freely flowing drinks. Someone with claustrophobia may be uncomfortable in a crowded, closed space. People with hearing loss simply can't hear very well in a bar. It's my feeling that any essential office functions should take place in the office. If showing up at the bar is necessary to be considered a team player, this is discriminatory. If you work as a beer wholesaler, the employer can fairly argue that sitting at a bar is an essential component of the job, but I can't think of many other examples. This is unintentional discrimination, but that doesn't mean it isn't discrimination.[82]

Company-Wide Meetings

Fortunately, most companies don't hold company-wide meetings frequently, but when they do, they're usually important and in large spaces like auditoriums. You should sit near the front. You may be able to hear the speaker, and if you're close enough, you may be able to speech-read as well. But you may not hear the questions from the audience.

If you have disclosed your hearing loss, you can ask to put your FM transmitter on the podium, or the speaker can wear a remote microphone that is paired with your hearing aid. But again, you won't be able to hear questions from the audience. And you may find it hard to ask the big boss to put your transmitter on the podium or wear a microphone when he's doing something like announcing mass layoffs or his own resignation.

The burden for this kind of accommodation should fall on the company itself, and the accommodation should be available whether or not the company thinks it has any deaf or hard of hearing employees. Almost certainly, the answer is that it does.

If you are upper management and running a big meeting, assume that one-fifth of those you are talking to are not going to be able to hear you clearly. Hire a CART operator and an ASL interpreter for these company-wide meetings. When someone asks a question, ask her to stand up, identify herself, and then repeat the question into the microphone. Otherwise those with hearing loss won't even know which direction the question is coming from, much less what was asked.

We—those of us with hearing loss—should ask for accommodations. But sometimes we don't. When I was still at the *Times*, there were two annual meetings open to the whole staff. One was the publisher Arthur Sulzberger's report on the health of the company. The other was a meeting held by the executive editor in which editorial employees could ask questions and air grievances. Then–Executive Editor Bill Keller called these "Throw Things at Bill." Sulzberger, in his own effort at just-folks collegiality, used to bring a stuffed moose to the meetings. It was supposed to represent the moose (elephant) in the room.

Even though several hundred employees would attend, there were no accommodations for people with hearing loss. The *Times* has a good record in hiring (and keeping) people with disabilities. It has a number of people who are openly and proudly part of the Deaf community on staff. How come no one thought to offer hearing assistance?

More important, how come none of us asked for it?

Discrimination's Gray Areas

Advocates for people with hearing loss urge disclosure as the answer. And often it is. But I want to mention just a couple of examples where disclosure was no help whatsoever. To be fair, though, nondisclosure probably wouldn't have helped, either.

The first was a young woman who told me about her experiences working at a nonprofit organization. She was well educated and well qualified for the job. In addition, she was open during the hiring process about her hearing loss. The woman who hired her was someone with whom she had previously worked on a project about hearing loss. Her hearing loss was progressive and as it got worse, she had increasing trouble talking on the telephone. She asked to be reassigned to a position that wouldn't involve so much telephone work, or for a captioned phone. Instead, her supervisor simply cut her duties. Eventually, her duties diminished to the point where she had almost nothing to do. She was then laid off, with the explanation that her job was not essential.

In a similar case, a young man who had worked at a tech firm was open about his hearing loss and was well qualified for the job he was hired for. But he couldn't schmooze with the others; he didn't go out to lunch or drinks. Eventually, he was fired, he was told, because collaborative thinking was important for his success in the job.

These are gray areas—not outright discrimination but instead a subtle undermining that eventually leads to grounds for dismissal. It's unlikely that either of these cases could have been won if the victims sued their employers for discrimination. Even though the explanations—that there was no longer a job for the young woman, or that the young man was not a team player—were clearly what attorneys call pretexts, it would be very difficult to prove corporate intention to discriminate.

The Odds Are Not in Your Favor

This is not to say there aren't many people with hearing loss who haven't done extremely well for themselves, becoming doctors and lawyers, professors and politicians, psychoanalysts and composers, and even professional football players (we in the HOH world love the Seattle Seahawks' Derrick Coleman).

Still, the unemployment statistics for the deaf and hard of hearing are shocking. According to a report prepared by Gallaudet University in 2011,[83] the unemployment rate for deaf and hard of hearing individuals aged sixteen and over was 16.1 percent. For hearing people the rate was 8.8 percent.

Breaking this down to those in their prime working years, the report, which in some cases relied on older information (2001, 1994) found that in the eighteen to forty-four age group, 82 percent without hearing loss were employed, but only 42 percent of those with severe to profound loss were. In the forty-five to sixty-four age group, only 46 percent of those with a hearing disability were in the labor force, compared to 73 percent of the hearing population.

Employment is related to education (as is income). The report also found, based on 2001 figures, that the national average for high school dropouts was 18.7 percent, but among those with severe to profound hearing loss 44.4 percent dropped out. For those who make it to college, 12.8 percent of the hearing population graduates, while only 5.1 percent of the deaf or hard of hearing population does. The number today for hearing people has gone up considerably, to a 59 percent graduation rate from a four-year college within six years. But the reading levels for deaf and hard of hearing—and thus college graduation rates—remain stubbornly low.

For decades, the mean reading level for those who grow up deaf or with severe hearing loss has remained stuck at the third-to fourth-grade level. It's hard to comprehend how this can still be true, but most experts on Deaf education agree that it is, and a recent report from another Gallaudet University professor confirmed it again.[84] For an interesting discussion of some of the reasons for this, I highly recommend Lydia Denworth's 2014 memoir *I Can Hear You Whisper*.[85]

Family income levels are about the same for deaf and hearing populations at lower income levels, but the difference becomes significant as income increases: In 2011, 29 percent of hearing families earned $50,000 or more, while only 14 percent of families with hearing loss did.

For those of us who want or need to work, who love our jobs, who want to succeed, hearing loss can undermine the best of intentions. Disclose or not? Damned if you do. Damned if you don't. But I hope these suggestions will help, and will inspire other ideas about how to make a difficult situation work as well as it can.

CHAPTER THIRTEEN

Mid-Career Hearing Loss, or, My Mistakes

*My mistakes were understandable,
but that doesn't mean they weren't mistakes.*

The vast majority of people with hearing loss in the workplace didn't start out that way. Their hearing loss probably came on gradually over a period of time, the result of noise exposure or aging. It can take a while before the affected individual becomes aware of the problem, and even longer before he or she is able to accept it. The timing of disclosure is affected by one's psychological journey to acceptance of the loss. That journey can take a long time. On average, people wait seven to ten years between first noticing a hearing loss and deciding to accept it and purchase hearing aids.

In this chapter, I'll talk about how my hearing loss affected me in the middle of my career. As you'll see, I made my fair share of mistakes. Maybe, you can learn something from them.

Bravado Works, Until It Doesn't

For the first decade after discovering my initial loss in 1978, I ignored it. For most of that time, I was working as a freelance magazine writer, which made it easier not to acknowledge any hearing problem. I wasn't in an office on a daily basis, so I wasn't at meetings or even talking much to people.

I wrote about archaeology and scientific fieldwork. My interviews often took place in the open air, in remote—and quiet—places like Turkey and Mexico. The interview subjects were often foreign, and so we spoke slowly, and repeated a lot. My hearing loss did not seem to be an issue. But others remember some hearing issues, and it embarrasses me to realize that even then some people saw through my pretense. In 1980, I spent a month in Antarctica researching an article for *The New Yorker*. Ira Flatow of NPR was there, too, and he later mentioned to my husband that he thought I'd had some difficulty hearing. I have no memory of it.

After I had children in my thirties, I no longer wanted to go on two- and three-week research trips, and my freelance career diminished. In 1988, *The New York Times Magazine* had an opening for an editor. I was a contributor to the magazine, and although I had no actual editing experience, I knew enough from being edited and from my early experience at *The New Yorker* as a copy editor to get away with seeming qualified.

I went in for an interview on a Wednesday with the managing editor and two days later I got a call asking if I could fill in for two weeks for someone who had just gone on emergency medical leave. The two weeks ended up being twenty-two years. I was formally hired six months later and at that point I had the mandatory physical that showed my significant hearing loss. I don't know if my bosses at the magazine were told about it, but it registers as just a blip for me in my early days at the *Times*.

I worked at the magazine for five years, thinking up story ideas, assigning them to writers, and editing copy when the story came in. It turned out that my instincts were right—I did know how to be an editor, even though I didn't have the résumé to show it.

In those years, I literally danced around my hearing loss. Walking with writers or other editors on the street, I moved around them so they were on my right, my good ear. Sitting at my desk, editing a story with a writer, we'd go through contortions so the writer was on my good ear side. I was open about it. It was a joke, even a kind of flirtation.

In 1993, I was promoted, a move that took me to the daily paper. Now the deputy science editor—the second senior person in the department—I often went to the Page One meetings to pitch stories for the front page of the next day's paper. These were daunting occasions, with the executive editor, then Max Frankel, and the managing editor, then Joe Lelyveld, at opposite ends of the table, grilling the editors about the stories they were presenting. I remember being nervous and hyper-attentive. I must have been a good lip-reader, because even then I was essentially deaf in one ear.

In 1998, I went back to the magazine, this time as deputy to the new editor in chief, Adam Moss. There was also a co-deputy, Gerry Marzorati, who had the title "editorial director." Gerry and I supervised the story editors and worked closely with Adam on all aspects of the magazine. We also edited many of the cover stories. I had a private office, so most conversations were held in a quiet environment. My right ear was still almost normal, and it was enough to sustain the illusion that I could hear.

In August of 2001, I turned fifty-four. The next month, 9/11 happened. We saw the second tower fall, many of us, gathered around the TV in Adam's office, and the world as we knew it changed forever. Journalism changed, too, and *The New York Times Magazine* with it.

After that, the pace ratcheted up as we quickly evolved from a features magazine to a news publication. The pace and pressure were relentless, with a backdrop of fear and anxiety. For the next few months, bomb threats and anthrax scares seemed to come day after day. Military personnel in full battle gear, armed with machine guns, patrolled the streets of Times Square and the subway stations. I had a fourteen-year-old daughter who took the subway to school every day, changing trains in Times Square. I worried about her constantly.

Our office was down the hall from the mailroom, and more than once suspicious envelopes brought men in full hazmat gear tromping past to the mailroom. We watched them go by, and wondered if we shouldn't also have some protection. We were issued gas masks, which eventually became never-used souvenirs.

Finally, my bravado and half-hearted attempts to manage my hearing loss had met their match: stress.

In the fall of 2002, we published a 9/11 anniversary issue, an ambitious and exhausting project that consumed us for months. Herbert Muschamp, the *Times*'s architecture critic, enlisted a prominent group of architects to propose a vision for a rebuilt downtown New York. The issue came together beautifully, but it coincided with a personal tragedy, when our designer, a young Canadian named Claude Martel, was diagnosed with cancer and died very quickly. We'd all thought his fatigue was like ours, a result of long days and nights working on the issue. (As for the visionary plan, Herbert Muschamp died in 2007, and his proposed downtown was never realized.)

My response to the months of intense work and then to Claude's death was to develop some flu-like symptoms, a ringing in my ears, dizziness, and nausea. It also seemed that I was not hearing as well as I had been. Eventually, I admitted I needed to see a doctor.

I didn't have an ENT. I asked a colleague for a recommendation and she sent me to Ronald Hoffman, then at Beth Israel and now at the Cochlear Implant Center of the New York Eye and Ear Infirmary. Dr. Hoffman found my hearing loss much more alarming than I did and ordered the same tests and treatment I'd had in 1978 and again in 1988 when I was hired at the *Times*: an MRI, tests for autoimmune disorders, the whole workup. He prescribed two weeks of high-dose steroids. He also recommended hearing aids—for both ears. The loss had progressed in my already damaged left ear, and I now had moderate to severe loss in my previously healthy right ear. I realized I'd been essentially deaf for months. Hearing aids were no longer an option. They were a necessity.

I still remember the mix of embarrassment and trepidation I felt when I told my boss, Adam, about my hearing loss and new hearing aids. I told him the truth, that I had an unexplained but serious loss. At fifty-four, I was beginning to feel old—I was in fact ten years older than Adam. I knew my hearing loss had nothing to do with age but I couldn't shake the stigma.

I worried that once Adam knew about the hearing loss he'd begin to think differently about my job performance. I kept up my daily bravado act, even after I got the hearing aids. The hearing aids helped, and I think he forgot I'd ever mentioned it. But this loss would have serious ramifications in terms of how I was perceived at the *Times*.

Disclosure: Once Is Not Enough

After the conversation with Adam, I never again mentioned hearing loss until I finally left the magazine in 2008.

Over this time, my hearing dropped in fits and starts. At one point, I got a new, stronger hearing aid in my right ear, and gave up wearing the one in my left because I felt it no longer helped at all. I was still able to talk on the phone fairly well with my "better ear," but I couldn't hear at meetings, and often I tuned out.

A few years later, when Adam left the magazine, both Gerry and I were candidates to replace him. I didn't understand until later, but it was a preordained decision. Gerry got the job. Realizing that I'd never actually been in the running was demoralizing and humiliating.

Was it my hearing loss? I knew it had affected my ability to jump into discussions and propose ambitious projects. I sometimes couldn't follow what was said and often was reluctant to speak up because I wasn't sure what others had said. But more important—and it has taken me years to realize this—I was working so hard to follow conversations and meetings that I didn't have the mental energy left over for thinking big thoughts and proposing creative projects. I was suffering from an overwhelming case of what neuroscientists call "cognitive load."[86]

In 2007, the *Times* moved from its old building on West 43rd Street to a new glass and steel tower. The interior was an open plan, surrounding a courtyard. The acoustics were terrible. I had a very hard time hearing in our glass-enclosed conference room, I hardly ever went to the big, noisy cafeteria, and even the elevators seemed to resonate. I scurried through the main lobby with its high ceilings and glass walls so I wouldn't have to talk to anyone. There was literally no place in the building where I could hear properly, not even in the small glass "privacy" conference rooms. Sometimes in frustration and exhaustion I would go across the street to the Hilton and sit in a big armchair in the lobby until I felt ready to face the office again.

By now, hearing loss was an undeniable presence in my daily life. I was not only stressed but also anxious and depressed. My confidence was undermined by the spurious search for a new editor for the magazine. I'd been an unwitting dupe in the effort to make it look like all avenues had been explored.

It was a chicken-egg situation. As my confidence plummeted, my hearing loss grew worse. Or was it the other way around? As my hearing loss plummeted, my confidence dropped.

I stayed at the magazine for another five years—in a more executive oversight role—each unhappier than the one before. I didn't have the hands-on editing work that I enjoyed and was good at, and that I didn't need my hearing for. I went to lots of meetings, which I did need my hearing for. The less I heard, the less I participated, the more depressed I got.

Here's what I should have done: As the parameters of my new job became clear, as the necessity to hear well became more and more a part of my work, I should have gotten out. I should have gone to management, explained my hearing loss fully and frankly, and asked them to find me a job that better suited my hearing abilities. I was a good editor, a good mentor, good with insecure and/or demanding writers. Those were all things that could be done with hearing loss, in one-on-one conversations. None of these were part of my job in those later years at the magazine.

An Excellent Opportunity, Blown

In the fall of 2008, I became the editor of theater and books coverage in the daily paper, editing theater reviews in Arts and Leisure and the weekly "Abroad" culture column.

When Sam Sifton, the culture editor, offered me the new job, I told him about my hearing loss up front—as well as my lack of knowledge of the theater community. He brushed both off as unimportant. And I think he immediately forgot about my hearing loss.

Although I was open about my loss, I failed to ask for appropriate accommodations before starting the new job. I had the chance to ask, and I still regret that I let it pass.

One accommodation, a captioned phone, would have made my life exponentially easier. As theater editor, I fielded dozens of calls from press agents every day: When were we reviewing their show? they'd ask. When would I like to see it, why weren't we reviewing it, how come I hadn't been to see it? I was used to pressure from public relations people, but I'd never experienced anything like this sense of entitlement.

The same was true of the books coverage, though at a lower key. Meeting with book publicists was part of the job. We always met in a small, closed meeting room, but even then the glass walls resonated, and hearing was difficult. I had the books in front of me, and I could tell which ones the publicist was talking about, but I couldn't understand enough to know exactly why, and what made it special.

I made errors. Once I discovered on a Sunday that I'd scheduled two book reviews on the same subject for the coming week. Anyone could have made that error but for me it was compounded by the fact that it took about six phone calls (on my then-uncaptioned home phone) to set things straight. It was very hard for me to follow what various people were saying, and they were all impatient at having to make a change on a Sunday. By the end of the phone calls, I was practically huddled on the floor with exhaustion, stress, depression, and doubt about my ability to continue in the job.

And of course there was the essential absurdity of someone with hearing loss being the theater editor. It didn't actually affect job performance: I could still assign ideas and spot new actors and know where the good stories lay. But I also went to the theater four or five nights a week, and even though I had great seats, I failed to understand most of what was said (or sung) onstage. I went because it was expected, and pretended to be enthralled. I did develop a love of theater, and today I go voluntarily but only to special performances for people with hearing loss, where there is a small screen with captions, thanks to the Theatre Development Fund.[87]

Two months into the job, the last week of October 2008, I got sick. It was similar to my 2002 illness—and like that one, it followed a period of immense stress.

At first, I thought I was having a bad reaction to a flu shot. I was dizzy and nauseated, my ears were buzzing. By the time I saw my ENT at the end of the week I was a physical and emotional wreck. The buzzing in my ears was so loud I couldn't hear what he was saying to me. He typed his questions on his computer for me to read.

We skipped the MRI this time, but once again he tried oral steroids. He also recommended a tranquilizer. I had started seeing a therapist a few months before, and she wrote me a prescription for Klonopin and a sleeping pill.

I didn't go to work that day, a Friday, calling in sick after the doctor's appointment. I spent the weekend in a panic, alternately enraged or in tears. On Monday, I went back to work, told no one what had happened, and tried to go on as usual. The buzzing receded. The new hearing loss persisted.

Now profoundly deaf in my left ear and with moderate to severe loss in my right, I continued to allude to the loss so obliquely that no one really understood what was happening to me.

The people I worked with closely knew I had some hearing problems. But that didn't stop them from engaging me in long phone calls that I could barely follow, in asking me questions from twenty feet away, in talking to me when I was focused on something else. I moved my computer so that I'd catch the movement of someone approaching in my peripheral vision, but I was still often oblivious of someone standing at my desk. One of my bosses in particular, a short woman I couldn't see above the computer terminal, who never announced her presence, always caught me unawares. I'd literally jump when I realized she was standing there.

I went through many more tests and treatments over the next few months, with no positive results. The following summer, I told my doctor I was ready for a cochlear implant. A couple of weeks before the surgery, I told Sam Sifton, the culture editor who had hired me, about the implant. His response was boyishly enthusiastic: "Cool!" he said. He asked me some questions about it. He seemed genuinely fascinated by the technology and for probably the first time in my life, my hearing loss seemed interesting.

Shortly after that, Sam was offered the post of restaurant critic for the paper, a job he jumped at. A new editor came into the department.

The Last Straw

I knew the incoming editor. He was someone I'd crossed paths with over the years, most recently in an executive training session where he'd paced around the room like a motivational speaker from hell. I was wary.

I decided to lie low for a while and see how he was going to run things. Meanwhile, my father was diagnosed with a recurrence of lung cancer after surgery the previous spring. We all knew it was a death sentence, though both my parents effortlessly moved into denial. Since I lived closest (by which I mean we were both on the East Coast, even if separated by six states and two plane trips) and also was the oldest, I was the de facto caretaker. I tried to set up a rotating series of visits, with my siblings. My sister, who lived on the West Coast and came when she could, said I was being bossy. (I was. Thank you, Tina Fey, for making that an endearing trait.[88])

In October, my cochlear implant was activated. A cochlear implant is pretty hard to hide—but I tried, yanking my hair over my ears, wearing scarves. I would have worn a hoodie every day if I could have gotten away with it.

In November, I got a curt note from the new culture editor about the performance evaluations I'd written for the staff I supervised. I'd been doing evaluations for years and never heard a negative word about them. Now I was being asked to rewrite every single one. The note made me uneasy.

I didn't do anything about the note until a few weeks later when a company-wide buyout offer was in effect. I needed a better sense of the new editor's plans for the department—and for me. When I went to talk to him, he responded with such venom about his plans, which included moving me out of the department, that I reeled out of his office in shock. When was he planning to tell me this? After the buyout, when I'd have lost the chance to retire with a nice package?

I was not a "team player," he said. I didn't tell him about my hearing loss then, either—it was too late to mend the misunderstanding. I was also so angry that I would have resigned on the spot rather than tell him. Instead, I dug in my heels and fought for my job for a week or so. But I couldn't continue working for him, and I didn't really want to move on to something new at the *Times*. I'd had enough.

By the end of the year, my two decades at the *Times* were unceremoniously over. I walked out—with a nice settlement, made nicer by my boss's obtuse behavior, which the company was forced to make financial amends for, beyond what I was owed as severance.

Learn from My Mistakes

For many of my former colleagues, my hearing loss remained a secret until my book *Shouting Won't Help* was published in 2013.

It took a long time to recover from my "retirement." It's not something I'd recommend for anyone with hearing loss. Once you've left an organization, particularly one where you've worked for most of your adult life, it's hard to get another job. Especially if you have severe hearing loss.

In the end, I think the answer is full disclosure. Do everything you can to keep that job. Ask for the accommodations due you under the ADA, and if that isn't enough, demand them. Keep a record of requests for accommodation that are denied or ignored. Speak up about incidents of unintentional discrimination. If you belong to a union, keep the union rep informed.

I was lucky. I'd been a writer before I was an editor, and I was able to go back to that. I still had my salary for a year, and I was eligible for a pension and Medicare in just a couple of years. Without severance, pension, and Medicare, leaving the paper would have been as disastrous financially as it was emotionally.

PART THREE

Travel and Leisure

CHAPTER FOURTEEN

Flying and Lodging

Plan for the worst and you'll find it's not so bad after all.

How ironic it is that just when you reach retirement age, have seen the kids through college, paid off the mortgage, accumulated a nest egg—just when you're finally ready for travel—your hearing loss may have worsened to the point where it gives you pause about embarking on adventures?

Put that worry right out of your mind!

Whether you're traveling alone, with a spouse or friend, or in an organized tour group, careful preparation helps ensure that you won't encounter obstacles to fully enjoying your trip.

This doesn't mean that things can't go wrong.

My twenty-seven-year-old daughter and I sometimes go on vacation together. Being the mother, I naturally gravitate toward being the boss and decision maker. Except when I can't.

In the fall of 2013, she and I went to Russia for two weeks. When we went to board our Delta flight at Domodedovo Airport in Moscow, we were turned away. The gate attendant spoke English, but airports are noisy and she had a strong accent. I had no idea what the attendant said and was completely dependent on my daughter to interpret for me. It turned out we'd overstayed our visa. We had filled out the application correctly, but the embassy had put the wrong date on it. The visa was in Russian, so we couldn't read it. That was no excuse, according to the authorities.

Over the next three hours, I trailed Elizabeth from one end of the airport to the other. We understood we were to ring the buzzer under a sign on a wall that said "Consul." It was "next to the shop that sells books." We rang, and waited. Eventually, an impatient woman appeared from somewhere down the hall, rather than from the door in front of us, and sent us to a third terminal to get cash from a specific machine, the only one the consulate would accept cash from. When we got back with the cash, we rang and waited again. I took a photo of my generally buoyant daughter sitting slumped on her suitcase, a picture of dejection.

We missed our Delta flight. The next one wasn't until the following day. We ended up on Aeroflot. Without Elizabeth's clearheaded calm and perfect hearing, we might still be in Domodedovo.

It was a very confusing situation: visa filled out incorrectly, incomprehensible and impatient directions from airline staff about how to extend it, huge airport, signs in Russian, little English spoken. I relied on my daughter to help. But if I'd been alone, I'd have thrown myself on someone else's mercy. If necessary, I'd even have traveled back into the city to the embassy and asked for help. Those snafus are incredibly annoying and pretty draining at the time.

My first rule for foreign travel is to have the address and phone number of the U.S. embassy in every country you're visiting. But that's just for last-ditch help. For all other situations, follow these general guidelines.

Be Prepared

I f you don't hear well, especially in a noisy environment, you don't want to leave anything to chance. You may have been a footloose backpacker following your whims when you were younger, but that's harder when you can't hear the answers to questions, often questions about directions on a noisy street or in a noisy airport.

Review all your travel documents before you leave, and make sure you have them all in one easily accessible place. Store copies separately—ideally, in the secure pocket or purse of a traveling companion. But if you're traveling alone, put them in a suitcase or bag different from the one where the originals are stored. Leave additional copies at home or with a friend.

These documents should include not only the obvious ones like your passport and plane tickets, but less obvious ones as well. Print out all your contact information—who you'll be seeing, where you'll be staying—in every city you'll be in. Print out every reservation—with confirmation numbers. Print out directions to every hotel. You're going to visit your daughter in L.A., whom you call every single week. Surelyn you wouldn't forget her phone number, right? Print it out just in case your phone dies. Don't rely on memory for anything.

Don't forget to bring extra batteries and a backup hearing aid or cochlear implant. Make sure all your luggage is clearly marked with your name and address. Don't pack anything crucial—hearing aids and batteries, medications, travel documents, etc.—in your checked bag. It's always good to have a pen and pad available in case you need someone to write down directions or information.

Finally, chargers. People with hearing loss generally have a lot of chargers: for their cochlear implant batteries, their phone, their laptop or tablet, their FM transmitter/receiver, their e-book reader, their camera. Don't forget adapters and a power strip to plug all those chargers in.

Tips for Flying

Did you print the confirmation numbers for each of your flights? Do you have your full itinerary readily available? Have you checked to make sure what terminal your flight leaves from?

I'm guilty of failing to do each and every one of these. I may print out an e-ticket before I leave, but it sometimes disappears between the house and the airport. It's a lot easier to get a substitute if I have written my confirmation number in my datebook, along with the flight schedule.

As for terminals, that info is probably on your ticket and it's important to note. It's not a disaster if you've left enough time to get from Terminal 3 to Terminal 5 when you realize you've made a mistake, but it adds to the stress. Riding the train to Charles de Gaulle Airport a few years ago, I realized that the train I was on went to one terminal and the departure gate was most likely at another. A very nice French businessman overheard me and my companion trying to figure out what we should do, and offered to help.

Where you sit on a plane can make a big difference in terms of comfort. For those with hearing loss, that includes sitting in quieter areas of the plane. In general, the back is noisier, as the seats are near the restrooms and galley. This is where you'll find people congregating and talking, brushing past you, maybe even dropping magazines or food, jostling your elbow as they go by if you're on the aisle. Many people don't like to make plane reservations online, but it's the best way to pick a good seat.

Sometimes you can't choose a seat when you reserve—some airlines wait until thirty days before the flight to open the seating chart to the public. Avoid those flights if you can. But if you can't, find out when the seating chart will become available and go online as soon as it's possible to choose a seat.

Seat Guru (seatguru.com) is an invaluable resource for information about seats. You can get the specifications on any seat on any major airline flight. It will tell you if the seat doesn't recline, if it has equipment blocking your foot room, if it doesn't have a window. It'll also tell you if the seat is near a particularly noisy area of the plane.

Airlines that use other carriers for flights (for instance a Delta flight to Paris might be operated by Air France) often will never show a seat chart. You're left with suggesting your "preference"— aisle or window—and often end up with neither. Somebody has to sit in those middle seats.

If you fly more than a few times a year, try to always fly on the same airline and join that airline's frequent flier program, which will entitle you to better seats. If you're flying overseas and an upgrade is available—usually labeled "economy plus" or something similar, at a cost of $100 or so—that will also ensure you more comfortable seats, closer to the front, where it's also quieter.

Will Your Cochlear Implant Set Off the Metal Detector?

I've never had a hearing aid or cochlear implant set off the alarm, although it may be possible if a detector is set to be especially sensitive. If you're worried about it, put your hearing aid or cochlear implant in the little dish provided for jewelry and other small valuables. Of course then you won't be able to hear anything the TSA says as you pass through security.

Boarding

Who among us—regardless of our hearing level—has not stood at a crowded airport boarding gate while an attendant shouted incomprehensible information about which zone was boarding next?

I've had several humiliating experiences, trying to wing it by guessing which zone is shuffling onto the plane. I've held out my boarding pass, hopeful and polite, and been curtly told that I was not in that particular zone and to go back to the waiting area. Worse, some airlines board back to front (like Jet Blue), some front to back.

It's hard to guess if Zone 5 is the beginning or the end of the boarding order.

Here's a tip: Before boarding begins, go up to the gate attendant and say you are hard of hearing and won't be able to hear the zones called. Nine times out of ten, you'll be told to go ahead and preboard. You'll never fight for overhead suitcase space again.

Once everyone is seated, tell the flight attendant or your seatmate that you are hard of hearing and ask him or her to please pass on any important information coming over the P.A. system. I figure the pilot is usually yammering about who's ahead in the Giants-'49ers game, but sometimes you really do need to know what he's saying.

Transportation Once You've Arrived

If you'll be traveling from the airport by public transportation, research in advance how much it costs and how you pay for it. New York City buses accept only a MetroCard or exact change. How do you get a MetroCard? In New York, it's from a machine, cash or credit. But it's different in every city that has a metro. I find Washington, D.C., especially confusing because the fares differ according to zone and time of day. How is a visitor supposed to know what zone her stop is in, or what constitutes "peak" in D.C.? (D.C. residents claim it's very simple.)

If you're on a bus or van, sit near the driver and ask him to tell you when you reach your stop (which you should have researched in advance). Know where you're going once you get off the bus.

If you're taking a light-rail connection, check the schedule in advance and make sure it's easy to find (if not, print out a map). Again, make sure you know how to pay for it.

If you're taking a taxi, research in advance how much it will likely cost. In some cities, airport to midtown fares are flat rates—but they don't include the cost of tolls and sometimes do include additional fees. Be prepared to pay in cash in case the taxi doesn't accept credit cards, and in local currency if you're in a foreign country.

If you're taking the courtesy shuttle to a hotel, make sure you know exactly which hotel you're going to. A year or so ago on a trip to San Francisco, I stood at the chilly, damp shuttle stop while one Hilton Garden Inn shuttle after another passed. I knew mine was the "airport" hotel but none of them said "airport." Did I want "Gateway Blvd."? Or was it "Burlingame"? Two others also breezed by several times. I tried the courtesy phone but couldn't hear. I should have had the hotel reservation in my bag with all my other documents.

It's taken me years of mishaps and humiliations to collect these strategies. Hearing loss is invisible, and it's best to be proactive to avoid difficult situations. I learn new things all the time.

Hotel Rooms

A hotel room can be a great luxury, but for the deaf or hard of hearing it can be frustrating and even dangerous. At home, you may have a captioned phone, you may have a bed shaker alarm clock, you may have a fire alarm system designed for the deaf and hard-of-hearing, you may have captions on your television. You'll need to find a hotel room that includes these features.

In the United States, hotels, motels, inns, and other places of lodging are required to have a minimum number of rooms that are accessible to the deaf. The one exception is a typical bed and breakfast—a building where the owner lives and has fewer than five rooms to let.

These hearing accessible rooms, half of which must also be accessible to people with mobility requirements, must provide hearing aid compatible telephones (phones that work with a telecoil), TTY service (though this is gradually dying out), visual and vibrating alarm clocks and wake-up calls, decoders for accessing closed captioning on television (although why the TVs don't have automatic closed captions is beyond me), visual and tactile alarm systems, and some visual indication that someone is knocking on the door. These hotels also have to provide assistive listening systems in meeting rooms, although they may claim it's the organization putting on the event that is responsible for the assistive listening system.

The ADA's Accessibility Guidelines for Buildings and Facilities requires that new and renovated hotels provide "at least 4 percent of the first 100 hotel rooms and approximately 2 percent of rooms in excess of 100 to be accessible to both mobility-impaired and deaf or hard of hearing individuals."[89]

Hotels are not required to provide interpreters, CART, or hearing loops at the check-in desk. Instead, the ADA allows the exchange of notes. For longer, more complicated exchanges, however, the ADA says the hotel must provide an ASL interpreter or CART services. For telephone conversations, the hotel must provide TTY service at the front desk and make sure someone is trained to use it. Service animals are permitted anywhere a guest can go.[90]

You will help not only yourself but also others with hearing loss if you ask every hotel you go to about accommodations. The more requests a hotel gets, the more likely it is to install ample accessibility equipment.

Until all hotels are compliant with the ADA requirements, it's best to ask in advance for a room with facilities for those with hearing loss. If you like to make your arrangements online, most of the major travel sites allow you to specify that you need hearing accessible hotel rooms.

On Hotel.com, Expedia, Travelocity, and other online sites, first you put in the search information for your hotel—the area and the dates. Then when the list of hotels comes up, look at the left-hand panel, where you can choose from "Neighborhood," "Landmarks," and so on. Click on "Accessibility Features" and you'll get a menu of options, including "accessibility equipment for the deaf."

Unfortunately, from there you'll probably need to call the hotel. The travel sites will tell you if an accessible room is available for your dates, but usually will not specify what kind of accessibility equipment is available. A person with hearing loss won't benefit from a Braille telephone.

Before I researched this chapter, it never occurred to me to ask for a hearing accessible room, but I will from now on. I used to have a "Shake-N-Wake" travel alarm, but I left it somewhere. When I finished writing this paragraph, I went online and ordered a replacement from Amazon.com for $16.99. You can wear it on a wristband.

Even with my Shake-N-Wake, though, I'll ask for a hearing accessible room next time I'm in a hotel. Why should I risk sleeping through a fire alarm or a loud knock on the door?

CHAPTER FIFTEEN

On the Road

Do you need a hearing aid to drive?

When I renewed my driver's license a year or so ago, there was a box to check off to indicate whether I "need" a hearing aid to drive.

What a moral dilemma!

I do need a hearing aid to do just about anything but sleep. I can't say that the hearing aid helps much with driving, though. The noise of my car—not one of those silent super luxury models—is so loud that I can't even hear the radio, much less understand what might be said on it. I sometimes listen to music, but all I hear is the beat.

For driving, I rely on my eyes. My eyes are shifting constantly from the rearview mirror to the side mirrors, all the while keeping the road ahead in view. If I pass another car or change lanes on a highway, I lean way over so I'll be able to see if another car is in my blind spot. I'd immediately be aware of an emergency vehicle coming up behind me, because I'd see it even if I didn't hear it. In fact, that has happened several times recently, when I was going just a bit too fast.

I didn't check off that box. I figured if I did, the Department of Motor Vehicles would in one way or other delay renewing my license. It might insist I get a letter from an ENT. Not a major effort for me, but a bother. Also, I figured, if the DMV really cared about hearing, it would require a hearing test just as it requires a vision test. Somehow, that box seemed like an empty gesture to the ADA. *Yes*, the DMV was saying, *we take hearing loss seriously*.

There's no law barring the Deaf or hard of hearing from driving—that *would* be a violation of the ADA. So why the question in the first place? In 2009, Neil Bauman began a column about driving with hearing loss this way: "'How do you drive if you can't hear?' is a question I've been asked a number of times. And I normally answer, 'I use my eyes when I drive. What do you use?' 'Judy,' a hard of hearing lady, responding to this same question, quipped, 'I use my hands. My ears aren't long enough to reach the steering wheel!'"[91]

No Distractions. Ever.

Even though there are no restrictions on driving with hearing loss, that doesn't mean you should take your ability to drive for granted. For most Americans, driving is as automatic as walking. You learn young, and you do it almost every day of your life. But if you have hearing loss, you have to compensate by a more vigilant use of your other faculties, in this case seeing. And if you have recently developed hearing loss, you need to train yourself to drive visually.

One important rule: No multitasking in the car. No talking on the phone, even a hands-free phone. No eating, especially sloppy sandwiches. Make sure your drink containers have the lid securely attached so that you're not distracted by coffee spilling in your lap. Have your radio tuned to the station you want before you move the car.

I assume that your kids will be safely strapped into child seats, but don't get involved in squabbles with them while you're driving. Pull over, turn around, and talk to them (or yell at them, or whatever the necessary response is) face-to-face. If you have hearing loss, you'll need to read their lips anyway. And face-to-face is a far more effective way of getting kids to behave. Besides that, trying to speech-read via the rearview mirror is going to give you a mirror image of the person's lips. You're not going to be able to do it.

Keep your pet in the backseat, seat belted. A simple harness clipped to the regular seat belt keeps the dog or cat from flying through the windshield if you stop suddenly but also keeps the dog from licking your ear or jumping into your lap. Many people (hearing and not) crate their dog or cat in the car. This is safest for both you and your pet.

If you have your eye on the road, you'll be attuned to brake lights ahead and be prepared to stop—or slow down. Who knows, it may be a speed trap anyway. You should notice the flashing lights of emergency vehicles as soon as they are in sight through the rearview mirror. If a highway patrol car gets to the point where it's right behind you before you notice it, you're not being vigilant enough.

Encounters with the Law

What if you're pulled over? This can be difficult and even dangerous for someone with hearing loss. Even if you tell the cop you have hearing loss, he's still going to expect you to answer his questions. Remember, you don't *look* deaf. "Lady, do you know how fast you were going?" The correct answer is not to reach over to the glove compartment for your registration.

This situation is even more difficult at night, when the head-lights from the police car behind you may blind you. What if the officer doesn't get out of the car but blares through his loudspeaker "Get out of the car!" Or was that "Don't get out of the car!" That kind of misunderstanding can get you killed, or at least roughed up. This is even more of a possibility if you also happen to be young, male, or black. In 2014, Pearl Pearson—a grandfather (with both a son and son-in-law in law enforcement), who is Deaf and black—was pulled over by a highway patrolman. When he failed to respond properly, the patrolman handcuffed him and put him in the police car. The incident was videotaped, and it is clear that he was treated roughly enough to require medical attention.

I first read about Pearl Pearson on Shanna Groves's "Lipreading Mom" blog.[92] The case got a great deal of attention among the Deaf and HOH community, and a fund-raiser was held to help with med-ical and legal expenses. The local law enforcement community also paid attention. Pearson had a note on his car visor saying he was Deaf, but unfortunately he didn't get a chance to show it before he was handcuffed and bundled into the police car. That visor message is something that all of us with hearing loss should have. You can download a copy and print it out from Google images.[93]

In her column on Pearson, Shanna Groves provides highly sen-sible advice, which I am going to quote:

"After getting pulled over and before the officer approaches your vehicle, unclip the visor message and place it over your steering wheel. Roll down your driver side window. When the officer stands next to your car, keep both hands on the steering wheel and say 'I am deaf' or 'I am hard of hearing.' The officer will also see your visor message in front of you. From that point on, watch the officer closely for visual cues on how he or she wants you to proceed. If you still do not understand the officer's words, repeat 'I am deaf (or hard of hearing). I did not understand what you just said because I couldn't hear you. Would you please write down what you just said?' If you are unable to speak, motion your head in the direction of the visor message, which will explain that you cannot hear."

As Groves and others point out, make sure this visor message is *on* the visor, not somewhere in your purse or the glove compartment where you're going to have to shuffle around looking for it. The ACLU and the actress Marlee Matlin teamed up to produce a video[94] on how to handle a traffic stop if you are deaf or hard of hearing. It has useful advice for both those with hearing loss and those who hear perfectly. Matlin uses ASL in the video, but it is also captioned and there is a voice-over for the hearing.

The invaluable Neil Bauman has also written about visor cards. He gives several other links to visor cards, including one you can order for $4.95 that is laminated. His 2005 column on visor cards[95] relates some alarming instances of people with hearing loss being pulled over and having their hearing loss misunderstood. Get yourself a visor card.

CHAPTER SIXTEEN

Dining Out

Noise was the number one complaint in Zagat's 2014 survey.

The bad news is that restaurants are noisy. The good news is that a few restaurant owners are finally paying attention. And the acoustics industry is taking up the challenge.

Five years ago, when I was researching my memoir, *Shouting Won't Help*, I found some scattered anecdotes about restaurant noise: Mario Batali likes Radiohead and Guns N' Roses in his kitchen at Babbo. Wolfgang Puck likes Led Zeppelin. I also found a few research studies on the effect of noise on diners. One 2008 French study found that turning up the music in a bar resulted in patrons finishing a beer three minutes faster than at a lower decibel level.

Noise was the number one complaint in Zagat's 2014 survey and has been for the past couple of years. And restaurants are responding. "Acoustics is bound to become the next big thing in providing a great dining experience," proclaimed a headline on a website devoted to controlling noise, called Elevating Sound.[96] Regional newspapers and city magazines have covered how local restaurants are attempting to dampen the noise. In 2013, *New York Magazine* food critic Adam Platt dubbed the preceding decade "The Great Noise Boom." It was clear he was ready for this trend to pass:

"Ask any weary gastronaut about the single most disruptive restaurant trend over the past decade or so," he wrote, "and they'll give you a succinct, one-sentence answer. It's the noise, stupid."[97]

A Little Background

What got us into this situation in the first place? It used to be that you went out to a restaurant to avoid the chaos and distractions of preparing a meal at home. If you were at an expensive restaurant, you sat in a hushed elegant dining room, with attentive waiters silently serving and removing plates when you were actually finished eating. (Not so today. Another big Zagat complaint is waiters who snatch your plate away before you're done.)

Adam Platt credits Mario Batali with the idea of taking the kind of music he liked and blasting it into the lovely dining room at Babbo. If noise is the single most disruptive trend, fashions in restaurant design over the past two decades all contribute to it: Restaurants have become more casual, with noisy bustle an important part of the ambiance. Spaces are often expansive, in converted warehouses or factories with brick walls and big windows and concrete or tile floors. Open kitchens are another widely adopted trend. Sometimes the kitchen is separated from the dining room by a glass or Plexiglas partition, a surface that bounces dining room noise back into the dining room. Sometimes the kitchen is completely open, so that the cooking clamor melds with that of the dining room.

The décor often picks up on the industrial style of the architecture, with brushed metal tables and chairs, set close together. Community tables in the middle of the room are popular, adding conviviality as well as noise. The bar and dining area are often contiguous.

Dividing the restaurant into smaller spaces is not only *not* the answer but often exacerbates the problem. As Platt wrote, "It's a snowball effect. You get a hundred drunk people in a small room and crank up the music, and soon they're screaming at the top of their lungs to hear each other. It's the perfect storm."

Food has become a national obsession, thanks to Chef TV, as I think of it, and the competitive chaos of the kitchen as an element of the dining experience. Upscale restaurants in cities like Boston, Austin, and Atlanta enthusiastically adopt the trends set by celebrity chefs. So do upscale restaurants in smaller cities—sometimes cities where you can't imagine there are enough people with enough money to fill the place. A couple of years ago, I had dinner in Lewiston, Maine, an old mill town now notable partly for the number of Somali immigrants who have settled there and partly for Bates College, a small liberal arts institution. The décor, menu, prices, and noise were all close to what you might find in a New York restaurant. It was tasty. It was noisy. And it was packed.

Quiet Conversation?

In 2014, Zagat published a list of "quiet conversation" restaurants. Most were very pricey—Le Bernardin at $162 per person was number one (and number one in Zagat's "best food" survey). Second on the list was Chef's Table at Brooklyn Fare ($321 per person). Lower down on the list there are more reasonable choices, with an Upper West Side neighborhood favorite, Henry's, clocking in at $39 per person. I eat there a lot and it can be quietish, but it depends on where you sit and how loud the neighboring tables are.

How you hear in a restaurant has a lot to do with your individual hearing and also with the kind of correction you have. If you have untreated hearing loss, you're not going to be able to hear in a noisy restaurant because the ambient sound drowns out voices. But you're probably not going to find it painful—at least not literally painful.

Those of us with hearing aids and cochlear implants also can't hear our tablemates (unless we use assistive technology; more about that later), but we *are* hearing every noise in the restaurant amplified by our devices. It sometimes *is* literally painful. That's why so many people take off their hearing aids in restaurants. It alleviates the pain, but it doesn't increase the ability to hear the conversation.

That said, I've had dinner with friends at hearing loss conventions—people who wear hearing aids—in restaurants where they seem comfortable and yet I can't make it past the appetizers. I'm more sensitive to noise than some.

My hearing family members in their twenties and thirties seem to have no problem. (Maybe they're already going deaf from all that iPod listening, despite my constant haranguing to turn it down!) My husband and I sometimes have dinner with them in their favorite Brooklyn neighborhood places. Fun, but primarily a taste and visual experience—not a listening occasion.

Get the Right Table

I've learned—from experience, and from friends—how to optimize hearing when eating out.

Before you even make a reservation, Google the name of the restaurant and "noise." That will give you an idea if the food and décor are worth sacrificing conversation for.

Space between tables, acoustic tiles on the ceiling, curtains on the windows, and tablecloths are all a good sign. So are booths. One Upper West Side restaurant, now closed, had a long upstairs room with a window overlooking Broadway. The room had a bar (always noisier than tables) but the window had a heavy velvet curtain. If I sat with my back to the curtain, practically enfolded by it, I did quite well. That was the only seat in the restaurant I could tolerate.

Most people with hearing loss know they will do better if they sit in a corner, with their back to the wall. The same thing is true of sitting in a booth, as long as the back of the booth is higher than your head. My neighborhood diner has booths, but they're only shoulder high and so all the noise from other diners and the kitchen and the busing station floats into your ears unimpeded. You also need good lighting.

Speaking of the busing station, don't sit anywhere near it. The clatter of plates and cutlery will drown out everything else.

Avoid banquettes. They're comfortable, but the tables are usually close together and it's hard not to overhear conversations on either side of you. If there's a banquette table open and the diners on either side look like they're on dessert, you can take a chance that they'll soon be finishing up, leaving you and your dinner mate in blessed isolation. But that's a gamble, because you never know who will replace them. Always avoid sitting next to a party of four or six at a banquette table, especially if they're businessmen. (Businesswomen, in my opinion, tend not to be so loud.) The more people at the table, the louder the conversation.

Don't sit near the bar. Not only will you be near people drinking, laughing, and talking loudly, there may also be a television, and there will inevitably be music. In bars, the background music tends to become foreground, even if the restaurant itself is relatively quiet.

Sometimes the purpose of the restaurant is the music—a jazz bar, a country music barbecue joint—with food secondary to listening. Sometimes, though, the live music is meant to be soothing. There's a restaurant I like that's big and relatively quiet, with spaced-out tables and a separate bar area. I went there for Sunday brunch recently. The crowd was smaller and quieter than at dinner, but there was a trio playing soft jazz and standards, and I couldn't hear a word over it.

Outdoor dining can be a good solution, but it depends on the location. In my neighborhood, the Upper West Side of Manhattan, the outdoor dining spaces tend to line the north-south avenues: Broadway, Amsterdam, and Columbus. All three are heavily trafficked routes. At night, eating outdoors at a Broadway cafe, the traffic is downright entertaining, but not conducive to conversation. You see eighteen-wheelers going by with pre-poured reinforced concrete barriers or fifty-foot steel Jersey beams. If it's around the time of the annual boat show, you see one yacht after another seemingly sailing down Broadway. Car-carrier trucks also use Broadway, giving you a preview of the coming automobile season. In fact, most anything large going to midtown or downtown Manhattan takes this route, because the highways are closed to commercial traffic. The popular street artist Banksy's pig truck drove by one evening.

Some restaurants have patios or gardens in the back, and in general it will be quieter there, unless it's also where the air-conditioning unit for the building is situated. Trees and trellises help baffle sound. If you've ever eaten in an outdoor café in a Mediterranean country, with a grape arbor overhead, you've probably experienced acoustic heaven, as far as dining is concerned.

Rooftop restaurants, as I've discovered to my dismay, can be very noisy, especially if they're near a highway. Those fabulous spaces in downtown Manhattan with terraces overlooking the Hudson also overlook the West Side Highway. They're loud.

Online reservation services like Open Table allow you to include in your user profile the request for a quiet, well-lit table. The request will usually be accommodated.

Finally, if you want a quiet restaurant, eat early in the evening and early in the week. I know, I know ... it's beginning to sound like the early bird special.

Making a Quiet—but Not *Too* Quiet—Space

The fact is that a quiet restaurant, if it's too quiet, is going to have its own problems, whether or not you're using corrective devices. You'll be able to overhear the conversations of neighboring diners. The phone ringing at the front desk will sound like an alarm clock. A chair scraped along the floor will be as grating as fingernails on a blackboard.

The trick—at least for restaurants where people want to talk to each other—is a friendly background buzz. Restaurant designers call this "convivial intimacy," and the idea is to make guests feel secure in their privacy but also part of a larger whole. The easier fixes include the use of sound-absorbing materials like carpets and upholstery, wall coverings and curtains, and strategically placed acoustic panels. Acoustic tiles on the ceiling are especially helpful. But carpets and curtains may not have the vibe that a hip restaurant is looking for, and that's when the sound engineers need to be brought in.

Ideally, a sound engineer will be part of the original planning of a restaurant, because retrofitting a space can be much more expensive than doing it right in the first place. Sometimes it may involve rearranging a major architectural component. At a Mexican restaurant in Somerville, Massachusetts, the noise turned out to be so loud that the owner first moved the bar from the entrance to an adjacent space and then hired a soundproofing company to install acoustic panels on the walls and ceiling. The panels are two inches thick and fire retardant. The overall cost was $30,000.

Soundproofing is becoming increasingly sophisticated. Meyer Sound Laboratories in California, which manufactures loudspeakers and multichannel audio show controls, has also made a foray into restaurant design. Its first project was Comal, a big, bustling Mexican restaurant in Berkeley. Meyer Sound installed its Constellation technology. Designed for concerts and other events, it uses a combination of microphones, speakers, and computer digitalization that the owner or manager controls on an iPad.[98] Soundproofing material includes recycled jeans.

Comal's owner is the former manager of the band Phish, so it's not surprising he turned to innovative acoustic technology when thinking about sound levels at his restaurant. The iPad readings allow him to adjust the acoustics depending on the time of day or the size of the crowd. Soundproofing materials blend in with the industrial chic décor. One large panel, displaying a print by photographer Deborah O'Grady of a street in Oaxaca, Mexico, is part of the acoustic system. The *San Francisco Chronicle* reported that the system costs between $10,000 and $100,000,[99] with factors like space and materials accounting for the variation.

Recycled jeans were also used in a Toronto sports bar as sound-baffling material. Because the bar was retrofitted after it had already opened, the cost was high: $200,000, according to an article in *Restaurant Development and Design*. The noise levels came down from "dangerous" during big games to merely loud. The owner claims table conversations can go on despite the fan noise. I'm sure that's somewhat subjective. Not everyone agrees on what a friendly buzz is exactly, and as these soundproofing strategies show, it's not always easy—or cheap—to achieve.

Clark Wolf, president of a New York–based food and restaurant consulting firm, told *Restaurant Development and Design* that optimally the noise level in a restaurant should come in right under the one-on-one conversation level.

On the other hand, chef Alex Stupak who owns Empellon Taqueria and Empellon Cocina in New York, says that "when it's eight p.m. on a Friday and I can hear people's voices over the music, then you need to turn it up." He finally succumbed to pressure and soundproofed the Taqueria after it opened, adding a $60,000 cost that would have been lower if the soundproofing had been part of the original construction.[100]

Chef Ethan Stowell, who owns nine popular and critically praised restaurants in Seattle, is unapologetic: "I like a loud restaurant. I just do," he told a Seattle audience in 2012. "An individual customer might say, 'Oh, it's loud in here,' but a quiet restaurant is definitely not what you want."

Speak for yourself, Ethan.

CHAPTER SEVENTEEN

Parties

When nobody can hear, the playing field is leveled.

You Might Even Hear *Better* than Others

Few people can hear at a noisy party, whether they can hear or not. With my ability to read lips and with my cochlear implant set on Zoom, I actually do better at noisy parties than most.

When I add my FM system, I'm unbeatable! An FM system, as you will find in the next chapter, is a small two-part device consisting of a transmitter and a receiver that works with the telecoil in your hearing aid or cochlear implant to deliver sound straight to your brain by way of your ear (or at least it feels that way). The signal is picked up by the microphone worn by the person who is speaking to you, and you hear it very clearly because it is louder than the background noise and easier to hear over a distance. The key for those of us with hearing loss is to make the speech louder than the noise, as this means it will be less distorted and easier to understand.

You hold the microphone up to the speaker as if you were Ryan Seacrest interviewing Sandra Bullock on the red carpet. It should be set to the narrowest mode so it will pick up closer sounds better, i.e., those that are three feet away or less. Add speech-reading and you're way ahead of the other partygoers.

Conversations tend to be one-on-one at a party, and face-to-face. This is good for people with hearing loss. But if turns into a four-way conversation I just back gracefully away. No way I can follow that one unless I'm pretty aggressive with my FM interviewer technique. Sometimes a friend will turn to me and say, "We're talking about…" But I usually can't understand it the second time around, either.

Drink helps. Some claim liberal amounts help even more. Alcohol lowers inhibitions and helps contain the self-consciousness many hard of hearing people feel. Not that I'm recommending drinking to excess. That has the opposite effect. The fuzzier your mind gets, the harder it is to focus on those conversations, and communicating with others can be fatiguing enough without adding alcohol to the mix. It's still going to take a lot of cognitive effort to follow a conversation, even if everyone else is reduced to your level.

You also have to watch out for monopolizing the conversation. It's a lot easier to do the talking than try to hear.

Trouble Spots

I do go to parties—to see friends, to see what people are wearing, to eat good food, to see fancy apartments, sometimes even to see famous people. But I don't usually stay long. The noise is overwhelming, and the effort to make conversation is exhausting, even with the FM device. A friend has a fancy new FM called the Roger Pen, a wireless microphone that I'll discuss in Chapter 18. He swears by it. But at the same time, I can tell that he can hear only one person at a time, not a general conversation, unless he passes the microphone from speaker to speaker, and even then he misses a lot. I'm content (for now) to smile a lot, give hugs to old acquaintances, eat some hors d'oeuvres, have a few drinks—and go home.

I have always had a hard time in social gatherings. When I was young, I thought it was because I didn't have much self-confidence, but as I got older I realized it was because I couldn't hear.

I was never quite sure what was going on around me—what had been said, what had been asked. I missed jokes—always.

Introductions have always left me befuddled. I never hear names and even when I ask again, I still don't hear them. Worst is when someone is introduced just by a first name, which is even harder to pick up because it has fewer recognizable sounds than a full name.

It's surprising how much not knowing the identity of the person you're talking to inhibits conversation. You don't know if you're talking to someone you should know, someone you actually do know but have forgotten, someone you know of—the husband of a friend, someone who works at the same place you do—or someone who's just arrived from Kuala Lumpur.

Try as you might to glean some hints from the introduction or the conversation already in progress, you can't hear that, either. I can't hear names even when someone spells them for me. If eventually I do get the name, it's been such a huge effort getting there that I forget it immediately. I love name tags. Alas, they are not standard at social events.

Then there's the reverse. I know the person, I even know her name. But unless the conversation is about the weather, I'm lost. The person has a new job. Where? Doing what? The person has written a new book. The title is? The subject is? The person is getting married. Yes! Mental fist pump. I recognize the word *married* but she's sixty-something. Is that really what she said? Oh well, take a chance on "Congratulations!"

I was—and remain—especially uncomfortable at gatherings that involve serious talk—where politics or social policy are discussed, where academic or intellectual issues are hashed over, where art and movies and theater are the subject. I rarely contribute, because I never know what's been said. Sometimes I don't even know what we are talking about.

The Exhaustion Factor

Even with the FM system, and even if I'm doing as well as others, listening and understanding is just plain hard work. It's probably work for hearing people as well, but for them it's just a party thing. For me, it's daily life. So I'm less likely to put up with it just for "fun." My tolerance for a noisy party is usually no more than an hour and often quite a bit less. I've been known to leave parties after ten minutes.

Some environments are not conducive to hard of hearing people no matter how well they read lips. A party with live music, for instance, is usually a ten-minute affair for me. A wedding reception with endless toasts would be a ten-minute affair except that it's hard to duck out of those things. A particularly resonant party space, whether it's someone's living room or a cavernous restaurant, sets up too much competing noise.

My party tolerance is based on the ratio of how much I hear to how hard I've had to work to hear it. It's also a measure of how worth it that effort is. It doesn't take many muddled-through conversations before the effort outweighs the reward.

And then there's the exhaustion factor. The harder the work, the more quickly I get tired. Also the harder the work, the more I seem to drink, which further accelerates the pace at which I wear out.

Make It Easier on Yourself

There are a few ways to make parties easier:

Invite someone to sit on a couch with you and chat one to one. Not only will the couch provide a little acoustic baffle, but the noise will be above you, and less intrusive.

Stand near someone you know has a loud and clear voice.

Make sure the light is not in your eyes or, alternatively, that it's not too dark.

If it's a warm evening, invite the person you're talking with to go out into the garden or onto the terrace (though not if the terrace overlooks the West Side Highway).

The older I get, the more confident I feel about just standing to one side at a party, watching the chatter, nibbling the food, having a drink. And then I head home to my captioned TV show or a book.

PART FOUR

When Hearing Aids Aren't Enough

CHAPTER EIGHTEEN

Roger and Me: Assistive Technology

I can hear you, but I can't understand you.

How is it, you may be asking yourself after reading this far, that people with hearing aids still have so much trouble understanding what they're hearing?

They've spent their six thousand to eight thousand dollars, they've been back to the audiologist for fine-tuning, they wear the aids all the time. And they still can't understand what the lecturer on the podium, the actor on the stage, the eulogist at the funeral, or even the person across the table at dinner is saying. They can hear them. But they can't understand them.

People with mild to moderate hearing loss need amplification, and hearing aids are good at providing that. But when the hearing loss becomes more severe, several things conspire to make speech comprehension a challenge.

A 2010 survey of hearing aid wearers[101] found that the majority of consumers have "significant problems with the sound quality of modern hearing devices." Only 36 percent reported that they were satisfied with the performance of their hearing aids in noisy situations. Just 43 percent were satisfied with their ability to hear quiet sounds and only 44 percent felt comfortable around loud sounds. In other words, in each of these categories where hearing aids are needed the most, *more than half and sometimes more than 60 percent were not getting a satisfying performance from their hearing aids.*

A second obstacle to understanding is the pattern of noise-related and age-related hearing loss—the most common causes of hearing loss. These tend primarily to affect the higher frequencies, those between 1,000 and 6,000 hertz. These frequencies are where many consonant sounds are found:

Ch and *sh* register at just below 2,000 Hz, making it hard to tell the words *shoe* from *chew* or *chop* from *shop*. Making matters worse, these sounds look the same on the lips. They are also very soft sounds, so even people with mild hearing loss may not hear them.

At a slightly higher frequency you get *k*, *f*, *th*, and *s*, which are also very soft sounds.

Clustered between 1,500 and 2,000 Hz are *p*, *h*, and *g*. Add these sounds to the ones just below 2,000. Was that *chip* or *hip*, *wish* or *which*? These consonants sound alike to me whether they're at the beginning, middle, or end of the word.

Put these nine sounds together any which way with any of the five vowels and you're going to have a hard time distinguishing the "sinking ship" from the "stinking shit" from the "shrinking shift" and so on. The combinations are limitless. That's why looking at the speaker and watching the shape of the lips is important, as is understanding the context.

You probably will get the middle of the word—*ink*—but not the beginning or the end. This will be true for anyone with a mild to moderate *uncorrected* hearing loss. Unfortunately, it will also be true for anyone with a severe to profound hearing loss even when corrected, because the human ear is much better at detecting shifts in frequencies within sounds and words than a hearing aid or cochlear implant is. This is especially true at a distance, or when competing with other noise.

So what exactly does "at a distance" refer to? Unfortunately, the useful range of a hearing aid microphone (worn in or behind the ear) is six to eight feet. This doesn't mean you won't hear sound more than eight feet away, but you may have trouble deciphering that sound. Then add the interference of a couple talking loudly at the table next to you, or the choir singing softly as the preacher intones, overlapping background sounds on TV, or the air conditioner humming in your therapist's office—and you're going to find yourself saying "What?" a lot.

"The real problem with hearing aids," says Barbara Weinstein, founding executive director of the Doctor of Audiology Program at the CUNY Graduate Center, "is that the microphone is at the listener's ears and not at the mouth of the speaker."

If you find yourself facing some of these challenges, your audiologist may say you need a new and stronger hearing aid. (And you may.) But there are many technologies to boost the sound and clarity of your existing hearing aid, and they're a lot cheaper than a new one. This chapter will provide an overview of these assistive listening devices (ALDs). You can also find a good general discussion on the websites for the NIDCD (National Institute on Deafness and Other Communication Disorders)[102] and Sound Strategy.[103] Sound Strategy, the creation of assistive technology expert Cynthia Compton-Conley, offers useful and very comprehensive tutorials. Compton-Conley may be the world's foremost expert on assistive technology for people with hearing loss. She is a retired professor of audiology and director of the Assistive Devices Center at Gallaudet University. She is now the director of Consumer Technology

Initiatives at the Hearing Loss Association of America. Her descriptions on Sound Strategy are far more detailed than I have room for here, and I highly recommend the site.[104]

Telecoils

If you don't already have a telecoil, you can start by asking the audiologist to install one into your hearing aid. A telecoil, usually called a T-coil, was originally known as a Telephone Coil, because its primary use was to allow you to hear on hearing-aid-compatible phones. It's an inexpensive, small component in most hearing aids and all cochlear implants, and it gives you access to some important technologies both inside and outside of your home. Much like an antenna on old-fashioned televisions, the telecoil expands the functionality of your hearing aids and cochlear implants by delivering customized sound from the sound source. Many hearing aids include an "MT" setting on the telecoil so both the microphone and telecoil can be active at the same time and you can hear your husband talking to you while you're also trying to talk to a friend on the phone.

Why don't all hearing aids have telecoils? Audiologists don't always recognize their usefulness and may neglect to either order the T-coil or activate it. You should also be able to manually activate and deactivate your telecoil depending on the situation, such as turning it on when you're in a looped venue. A 2014 *Hearing Review* study found that 71.5 percent of hearing aids sold have a telecoil.[105] All cochlear implants have telecoils, but again there should be a manual option to switch to telecoil mode when you're in an environment with a hearing loop.

A telecoil is a small copper-wire coil inside the hearing aid or the processor of the implant. The user accesses it by pushing a button on the hearing aid or a remote. The coil interacts with wiring on the telephone's handset (or with a cell phone) to convert the phone's electromagnetic signal into sound inside the hearing aid. The reception is not only louder but clearer. The FCC requires "hearing aid compatibility" (HAC) for all "essential" phones, including most landline phones, and all phones manufactured in the United States.[106] Most office phones are hearing aid–compatible, but some models may work better than others to eliminate interference and facilitate clarity.

Many (but not all) cell phones are also hearing aid–compatible,[107] as I mentioned in Chapter 12. The FCC requires wireless phones to have a rating indicating hearing aid compatibility: M (microphone) and T (telecoil). To be labeled HAC, the phone needs a minimum rating of M3 and T3. M4/T4 is excellent.[108] When I bought a new phone recently, I spent quite a long time in the store trying different phones with and without the telecoil activated. I bought the one that had the clearest signal and the least interference.

ASHA,[109] HLAA,[110] and other sites offer guidelines on how to choose a hearing aid–compatible phone, including what to look for in the technical description. It's also a good idea to try them out in the store first, because everyone's hearing is different, and the phone that works well for me may not work well for you.

Some cell phones, despite having telecoil connectivity, will still buzz when you bring the phone to your ear. This is the case whether the telecoil is activated or not. Some but not all phones have circuitry to limit this interference. For this reason, many people use hands-free streamers when talking on the phone (see the sections on FM systems and Bluetooth).

The telecoil is also necessary if you want to use your hearing aids or implants with the three main large-area listening systems used in many theaters and concert halls. These are infrared (IR), FM, and induction loops.

Infrared devices pick up a signal beamed in a straight line from the direction of the stage. They work well for people with mild to moderate loss, who use a receiver and headphones. For many people with more severe hearing loss, these devices aren't enough. If your hearing aid has a telecoil, however, you can plug a device called a neckloop into an IR receiver worn around your neck, which will send the signal to your hearing aid. Your hearing aid will help process the sound custom tailored for your hearing loss. In addition, the sound quality will be much improved, simply by bringing the sound directly to your ear.

Infrared can be installed as a true stereo system, with the sound balanced as it would be in normal hearing. Cynthia Compton-Conley notes that if the user is wearing earphones, he or she can hear in true stereo, provided that the miking (or recording) of singers and musicians is properly done. She added, in an email to me, that if these systems are properly installed and maintained, they can be as effective as a loop system (the subject of Chapter 20), provided the particular infrared receivers are powerful enough to meet the listening needs of people who have more severe losses. Unfortunately, as she notes, the user has to borrow a receiver to access the system—theaters normally give them out at a concierge desk in the lobby, in exchange for a driver's license or credit card as security. Many people would rather not hear properly than acknowledge their hearing loss so publicly.

Many theaters and courtrooms install the infrared system instead of looping for a variety of reasons. For example, infrared signals cannot pass through walls, so they are used in courtrooms, where confidential information is often discussed. They are also used in buildings where competing signals can be a problem, such as classrooms or movie theaters.

Captions

Captions are probably the most universally available assistive listening devices. They not only substitute for sound but they can also make your hearing seem more precise. If I hear a sentence and see it written out in simultaneous captions, I will actually *hear* the sentence better.

Captions are available on most network and cable TV shows. You go to the settings menu and look for closed captions, or CC. ("Closed" simply means they're invisible until you activate them.) You may have a choice of CC1 or CC2. These usually indicate different languages. Try CC1 first, unless you want Spanish.

Some televisions, especially those with satellite or cable access, are more complicated. Basically, it's trial and error. But once the captions are activated, they should stay on until you actively turn them off. My TV remote has a captions button on it, and it's very easy to switch back and forth. In Europe there's no distinction between captions and "subtitles," but in the United States captions are for the hearing impaired and subtitles are for translating a foreign language. If you are using closed captions and then the movie or TV show decides subtitles are necessary for one reason or another, you'll have both, often overlapping. Annoying.

The captions on live TV—network news, game shows, and so on—are usually not as accurate as the captions on prerecorded TV. In fact a lot of them are hilariously bad. Network news broadcasts often can't even get their correspondents' names right. NBC's Richard Engel comes out Chard Angle. HLAA and other consumer groups have asked the Federal Communications Commission (FCC) to rectify this.

YouTube, TED Talks, and many online videos have a small button in the lower right-hand corner that allows you to turn on captions. Most movie and TV DVDs have a caption option. So does streaming on Netflix.

Increasingly, as a result of pressure from the FCC, movie theaters are offering personal captioning devices. There are different models. AMC theaters offer a small screen attached by a flexible neck to a rubber weight that fits in the cupholder. The screen shows two or three lines of caption at one time. The neck is long and the rubber weight is heavy. When I carry it from the concierge desk into the theater, I feel as if I have ET cradled in my arms. Regal theaters use special glasses that show captions, which some people prefer, but I haven't personally tried these. Both systems allow you to watch the screen and the scrolling captions simultaneously. Again, the combination of sight and sound makes for a more comprehensible experience. I would much prefer to have a small handheld captioning device. I don't know why theaters have gone for such complicated systems instead.

What about live theaters? Some are looped. The Theater Development Fund sponsors showings of Broadway and off-Broadway shows with a small caption board to one side of the audience, usually in the orchestra. (Through its Theater Access Program it also offers accessibility to the blind and those with other disabilities.)[111] Even if a theater is looped, however, some people have a hard time following dialogue or lyrics without captions as backup. Captioning is essential for me, but also for the deaf who use sign language and any other people with hearing loss who do not have hearing aids or other devices.

CART (Communication Access Real-Time Translation), which I have mentioned in several contexts, is one of the older technologies and offers a live-captioned transcript. Early CART providers had often started as court reporters, and the technology is similar. But a court reporter takes the equivalent of shorthand notes and then transcribes a full transcript later. A CART provider produces a full transcript in real time, as the discussion unfolds.

The CART captions are viewed either on a computer screen or, in a larger group, on a portable screen or a blank wall. CART is mostly used in larger groups. Like ASL, it's a form of hearing assistance that should be provided wherever people needing hearing assistance are gathered.

Some business and universities and other institutions will provide a one-on-one CART operator if a student or applicant requests it. At a university, that CART operator will attend classes with the student.

FM Systems

Personal wireless assistive listening devices allow you, the wearer, to receive an isolated signal directly from the source, which could be a speaker, TV, or other device. For speaker-to-speaker communications, these include FM systems, which have been around for quite a while, as well as a body-worn 2.4 GHz transmitter that resembles (but is not) a Bluetooth system. The technology is discussed on Cynthia Compton-Conley's Sound Strategy website.[112]

FM technology works on a radio signal that is transmitted by the speaker (who is wearing a microphone attached to an FM transmitter). The FM signal travels across the room and is received by a small FM receiver around the hearing aid wearer's neck. The receiver picks up the signal from the transmitter and sends it directly to the listener's hearing aid, cutting out most extraneous noise.[113] If you do not have a telecoil, the receiver is paired with earphones, which you wear in place of your hearing aids. The message is sent through the earphones to your ears and brain.

The first time I tried an FM system was at a training program on assistive listening devices. The speaker (who was demonstrating the device) was at one end of a crowded room and I was at the other. I was wearing headphones to receive the signal. I could hear his voice perfectly, even though there were twenty or so people between us, all talking. It was like the ultimate walkie-talkie, except that the unit provided only a one-way transmission. I could hear and understand him, but he couldn't hear me. It could be turned into a two-way wireless system—with both participants wearing both transmitter and receiver. Ordinarily, the one-way transmission version is used for conversations in a crowded room with the speaker close enough so that he can hear your responses. It can also be used in a lecture hall by putting the transmitter on the podium. The signal range is about 300 feet.

The one-way conversation approach works in a lecture, but what about more interactive environments, like a classroom? FM devices were originally marketed for students. The teacher wears the microphone and transmitter, and the student wears the receiver. This gets complicated when you have other students—asking questions, sharing ideas—without transmitters. The teacher either has to pass them the microphone/transmitter or repeat their comments so that the student can hear what was said. Some classrooms use overhead microphones for the students.

Williams Sound offers a simultaneous two-way system, the Digi-Wave, which uses a 2.4 GHz transmitter. The technology is similar to Bluetooth but works on a proprietary protocol. It allows two-way conversation between people who both have hearing loss, and can also be used by four or even more people. It has other uses as well, including guided tours—especially when there's a tour guide and a translator in addition to listeners. See the Williams Sound website for additional applications.[114]

Another device that facilitates conversation between multiple people is the Etymotic Companion Mic. It allows for four-way transmissions, so four hard of hearing people can each hear one another. Etymotic is about to come out with an upgrade, so you might be able to buy the old system on eBay.

A number of hearing aid manufacturers have their own proprietary FM systems, and users may well prefer one of these for a variety of reasons—the design, how easy they are to use, how the sound quality sounds to them. Being tech savvy is also a consideration: Some systems are just too complicated for some people.

Widex offers a family of FM devices, called SCOLA. In each system, the microphone/transmitter fits comfortably in the palm. The SCOLA Flex, for instance, can be used with other brands of hearing aids.

ReSound's FM device is a clip-on Unite mini-microphone that is used with the ReSound Up hearing aids. The Unite Mini Microphone and ReSound Up can be used as an alternative or as a complement to FM systems. Oticon has a variety of FM ear level systems known as Amigo, which are versatile and can be used with different styles and brands of hearing aids and cochlear implant processors. Amigo receivers are universal and can be used with nearly all other manufacturers' BTE hearing aids.

These are just a few of the options available, and new devices are coming out all the time. Cynthia Compton-Conley recommends the excellent blog "Federal Retirement," designed to aid U.S. government employees in retirement. Be sure to check out the section on hearing health care, "How to Manage Your Own Hearing Health Care."[115]

For the most part, FM systems are proprietary—that means you can't use a Phonak FM system with a Widex hearing aid without adding an extra device (at extra cost) to the hearing aid to act as a receiver. Eventually, the hearing aid companies will succumb to consumer pressure and standardize these devices. For now though, if you have a Phonak hearing aid and also need a cochlear implant, you should consider Advanced Bionics. Both are subsidiaries of Sonova and will work with the same assistive devices. You can also get an extra piece of hardware to link the two systems if they are different brands.

I bought Phonak's MyLink-SmartLink FM system after that demonstration a few years ago. At times it worked well, but it was a finicky device and some part was often not working. It's now being phased out in favor of Phonak's new Roger system.

Who, or What, Is Roger?

The Roger personal FM system seems to be the one all the tech geeks are putting their money on. It looks like a sleek pen and is one of the few pieces of hearing aid technology I've seen that has the visual and tactile appeal of, say, the newest iPhone.

The Roger Pen, a wireless microphone, can be worn around the neck by the speaker, held up to the speaker by the person with hearing loss, or placed upon a table. Additional pens may be added for group conversations where it is important that each speaker have his/her own transmitter close to the mouth to improve the listening experience. An optional clip-on microphone transmitter is also available.

Unlike FM systems (the Roger works on a digitally modulated, or DM, system), there's no need to wear an external receiver around the neck. Several types of receivers can be used, depending upon the listener's needs. One type is integrated into the hearing aid or cochlear implant. Another type has a universal connector so that it can be plugged into any brand of hearing aid or implant with the necessary jack. Finally, a reconfigured MyLink can be used by listeners using a telecoil-equipped hearing aid and/or implant.

The receiver transmits the signal to your hearing aid or cochlear implant, where it should be clear of extraneous noise.

Phonak also makes a Roger intended for teachers, the Inspiro. It's a clip-on mic. The student with hearing loss wears the receiver. Other students in the class can speak into a small handheld mic that works with the Inspiro system.

The Roger not only looks better than the old systems but the performance is by all accounts excellent. In one recent study, hearing-impaired people using the Roger were able to hear better in noise than normal-hearing people. That's quite a feat.

A 2014 article in the *American Journal of Audiology* by Linda Thibodeau, PhD, a professor at the University of Texas at Dallas, reported on a study conducted on the Roger, which was funded in part by Phonak.[116] The results were impressive. Using a test group of eleven adults with moderate to severe hearing loss who had been fitted with different brands of behind-the-ear hearing aids, and a control group of fifteen hearing adults, Thibodeau measured which group heard better in noisy situations. The people with hearing loss who used the Roger surpassed not only those using other FM systems (including others from Phonak) but the normal-hearing group as well. When the noise was turned up to 75 dB, the people with hearing loss using the Roger achieved 69 percent accurate word recognition, compared to only 7 percent by people with normal hearing.

In an interview published on Audiology Online,[117] Dr. Thibodeau discussed a model of hearing aid distribution that experts like Compton-Conley have been advocating for years. "Remote microphone technology should not be viewed as an add-on to a hearing aid," Thibodeau said. "For example, maybe you could offer three groups of options. Entry level one might be a clip-on microphone and basic hearing aids. Entry level two might be a Roger Pen to interface with cell phones, along with more sophisticated hearing aids. Entry level three might be for the person who is actively involved in group situations. This would include hearing aids, a Roger Pen and a clip-on microphone, or maybe hearing aids and a Williams Sound two-way system, with additional clip-on microphones. You could also suggest that they tell their family to purchase another clip-on for Christmas. Then, they can have multiple people with microphones in group situations, and hear interplay in conversations again."

Compton-Conley notes that what finally may make this distribution model a reality is the coming "hybridization" of products. Hearing devices can be sold along with other devices: a hearing aid and a streamer, for instance, or a hearing aid and FM system. This requires a thorough assessment of the patient's lifestyle and needs, budget, tech savvy, and other factors. It's imperative to find a good audiologist who has the training and is willing to take the time to provide you with what will most benefit you. "Look for an audiologist who doesn't focus solely on fitting hearing aids," Compton-Conley says. "That means one who embraces the wide range of technologies available to meet all your needs"—face-to-face, accessing media, telecommunications, alerting devices. The hearing aid, Compton-Conley says, is just one of many ways of addressing an individual's hearing needs.

If Compton-Conley's perspective is eventually adopted by the hearing aid industry, it will radically change the way we view hearing correction. "The mistake that the hearing enhancement industry has made is to focus on the hearing aid as *the* solution for everyone's listening problems," she wrote to me in early 2015. This focus, she went on, "may account for the historically high hearing aid return rate of 17 to 23 percent. The focus should be on each patient's hearing needs, which are influenced by his or her lifestyle. There are many ways of addressing an individual's hearing needs. Careful needs assessment can then be leveraged to properly inform technology choice. By using this approach, it will become clear that some people do well with hearing aids only, whereas others may need hearing aids plus other assistive listening technologies.

"And some people may not need hearing aids at all," she went on. "They may prefer to use assistive listening devices in selected difficult-listening situations. The need should drive technology choice, not the other way around." Compton-Conley's view is in direct opposition to the industry's traditional view.

Thibodeau compared buying hearing aids to buying a new car: "When you buy a car, you decide on your features up front. You don't take the car home and then add features later on. The dealer describes the features to you and you make a decision based on your needs—do you want the anti-lock braking system? Do you want the upgraded sound system that adjusts its level based on road noise? I appreciate the salesperson that explains these features and makes recommendations based upon my needs."

Friends who have the Roger are pleased with its performance, for the most part, though some say it's difficult to pair with your hearing aids. I've hesitated to buy it. I lose five regular pens a week and I worry I would also lose the handsome Roger in a very short time. It's also expensive. The list price for the full-featured pen is $1,017.50. There's a less expensive model called the Easy Pen. People who attend a lot of business meetings may want two or more Roger Pens, to put on different areas of a conference table.

A friend who bought the Roger last year told me he ended up paying $2,236, even at a 40 percent discount offered by the provider. Here's the breakdown for his Pen, I Connect (the additional piece with the second battery compartment), Roger X (the FM receiver for his cochlear implant), and Roger 15 (the FM receiver for his hearing aid):

Pen: $1,017.50 list / $610 paid
I Connect: $260
Roger X: $1,138.70 list / $683 paid
Roger 15: $1,138.70 list / $683 paid

Without the discount, the system would have cost $3,554.90.

Even though his cochlear implant and hearing aid were made by Sonova (which owns Phonak), he still needed the external receivers because both devices were older models. The Roger was introduced in 2014.

Bluetooth

Bluetooth technology, like FM, is wireless. A Bluetooth-equipped device (a cell phone, laptop computer, MP3 player, etc.) is paired with a streamer. The streamer transmits sound from the device to the hearing aids or implant.

When my cochlear implant was upgraded after five years, I was offered a choice of accessories. I chose a streamer. It's called the

ComPilot and because I have a Phonak hearing aid and an Advanced Bionics cochlear implant (both made by Sonova), it works with both without any additional device.

Now I can hear music or recorded books on my iPhone when I'm out walking the dog, streamed wirelessly directly to my hearing aid and implant. I can also use it for the telephone. And best of all, because I do a lot of driving, I can use it in the car. One drawback is that the streamer's functions are limited. I had to choose whether I wanted the streamer to work as a Bluetooth transmitter with both my hearing aid and implant, or whether I wanted the streamer to connect only to the cochlear implant as a remote device for changing programs on it. I chose the former. But the controls on the cochlear implant are not that easy to use. I am considering buying yet another device, an iCom, to control the programs on the cochlear implant.

The first time I tried to use the ComPilot to stream a recorded book from my iPhone, I couldn't hear much. I was in the park walking the dog, and the streamed signal was overwhelmed by environmental noise. My audiologist reset the controls, so now the Bluetooth blocks 75 percent of the extraneous noise on the cochlear implant side, and 100 percent on the hearing aid side. This lets the music or book or a phone call stream in with very little competing environmental noise.

My audiologist was a little concerned that I wouldn't be able to hear what was going on around me, which is true. For driving it's not an issue: I can't hear anyway over the din of traffic or the noise of the car on a highway (especially a wet highway). I use my eyes. But now my ears have something to entertain them.

But I walk a lot as well, and I now use the Bluetooth only on the hearing aid ear and leave the cochlear implant at full volume. After a police car trailed me for some blocks in the park one day before I registered it was there, I realized I couldn't hear anyone or anything coming up behind me.

Confused? So am I. After I wrote this passage I got a Roger Pen, which I am still learning to use. I'll reserve judgment on how well it works until I figure out *how* it works. Despite my audiologist's instructions and instruction manuals, it's going to take a while to get there.

A Hearing Aid Built for Your Smartphone

Eventually technology will eliminate the streamer—the middle man—and allow the signal to go directly from a smartphone, say, to the hearing aid and implant. Apple already makes this possible, through software built into the iPhone. Two "Made for iPhone" hearing aids, manufactured by ReSound and Starkey, are getting a lot of attention. (Don't give up the telecoil just yet, though, as we'll continue to need them for a lot of the existing systems for some time.)

The ReSound LiNX hearing aid offers direct wireless connectivity to the iPhone, iPad and iPod Touch.[118] A feature called Live Listen turns the iPhone into a microphone in a noisy environment. The cost is approximately $3,000. (At the time of this writing, it required OS 7 or higher to work but that may change.) Adjustments to volume and programming are on the Apple device as well as on the hearing aid.[119] *The New York Times*'s personal technology columnist, Farhad Manjoo, raved about the LiNX in an April 2014 column, saying that even though he doesn't have hearing loss he would wear the hearing aids all the time if he could (I'm not sure why he couldn't). He also tried out the Starkey Halo, another iPhone-connected hearing aid. "For the first time, I had fine-grain control over my acoustic environment," he wrote, "the sort of bionic capability I never realized I had craved."[120]

Forbes's Anthony Wing Kosner, who does wear hearing aids, also wrote about the Made for iPhone aids, and focused on the Starkey Halo i110. "It is an interesting reversal," he wrote, "but in an age where we are listening to remote audio for hours a day, wearing hearing aids is actually a *convenience.*" Kosner noted that when you program the Made for iPhone hearing aids you do it on the iPhone, which means you gain visual feedback about the adjustments you're making, something that's missing when you're trying to turn the little dial on the hearing aid behind your ear.[121]

Smartphone Apps

No matter how versatile and sophisticated these new devices may be, sometimes the only solution to hearing difficulties is the written word. I have several late-deafened friends who cannot use hearing aids or cochlear implants, do not know sign language, and rely on reading lips. Some new smartphone apps allow them also to receive information instantly in writing.

These include speech-to-text apps on a cell phone or elsewhere, as well as live captioning for phones and teleconferencing. An iPhone app called Dragon Dictation can be used by someone with severe hearing loss in a one-on-one conversation. So can Siri, using the Notes feature.

The speaker talks into the iPhone using the Dragon Dictation app, then hands the phone to the hearing-impaired listener, who reads the captions and responds orally. It's a little clunky—and not always reliable, but it usually works. And it works better the more you use it because the device learns to recognize frequently used specialized words (like "hearing aid") and also the voices of people you talk to regularly.

Smartphone users also have a microphone icon on the phone that lets you dictate a text message. My iPhone also has an app for Voice Memos.

And of course you can always carry a pad and a pen and write notes the old-fashioned way. Even a pad and pen can be an assistive listening device.

Some experts, like Cynthia Compton-Conley, think smartphones will eventually be used as hardwired universal hearing enhancement devices. Others are already using smartphones as assistive listening devices. Richard Einhorn, the composer and sound engineer, uses an iPhone app called SoundAmpR and very high quality wired, in-ear earphones. The app picks up the signal, and the earphone delivers it to the ear and minimizes background noise.

Assistive Technology for the Home

Hearing assistive devices also include those I mentioned in Chapter 8, as well as alarm clocks, fire alarms, doorbells, and telephone ringers that light up. New devices are patented and come on the market every day. You can buy them at retail stores, online, through specialty distributors like Harris Communications, and often through your audiologist. Some of these are free or discounted through state providers, if you submit an audiologist's letter that you have hearing loss. The captioned phone is one of these, and one of the most common and most useful.

Fire alarms are essential for those who can't hear at night when they take their hearing devices off. They are not smoke detectors, so you also need conventional smoke detectors. The alarms respond to the signal from the smoke detector and emit a loud low frequency warning and flashing lights. If that's not going to wake you up, they can also be fitted with a bed shaker.

In New York City, the FDNY came to speak at our HLAA chapter meeting and distributed these devices (which can be bought but are expensive). If you belong to an HLAA chapter or ALDA, check with your local fire department to see if it offers the same service. For a more complete discussion of fire safety, and for information about devices, see Hearing Loss Help.[122] Sound Strategy also offers useful tutorials.[123]

Finding the Assistive Device That's Right for You

Feel dizzy just reading about the options? So do most people. This is one reason to work with a very good audiologist.

HLAA, recognizing the confusion consumers face, recently initiated a three-year plan, the Consumer Technology Initiative, to create a website and an online product directory that will serve as a clearinghouse for consumers, hearing health professionals, and health-care professionals. The site will disseminate information about current and emerging technology to consumers, and also communicate consumer needs to manufacturers.

Up until now, navigating the assistive listening device world has been difficult for even the most knowledgeable users. When I first got my FM system, my experienced audiologist couldn't figure out how to configure it to work with both my hearing aid and cochlear implant. She consulted the manufacturer, she consulted other audiologists, we experimented using trial and error. Error prevailed. Eventually, a Gallaudet professor offered the correct answer.

The Consumer Technology Initiative should make that arduous search for answers a thing of the past. The website and directory are scheduled to launch in June 2015.

CHAPTER NINETEEN

Read My Lips!

If you can't see the speaker's lips, you can't read them.

Technology is useful, but there are ways to improve your speech comprehension that don't include technology at all.

That no-tech solution is speech-reading, what we used to call lip-reading. Lips are still all important in speech-reading but we've learned that paying attention to body language and facial expression are also key elements in understanding speech.

When I went to see the much-acclaimed movie *Birdman*, with Michael Keaton, there were no assistive listening devices available. I decided to give it a try anyway.

From the opening scene, I knew it wasn't going to work for me. Michael Keaton speaks his first lines with his back turned to the camera (you can see that scene in the trailer). In subsequent early scenes, the speakers are in profile. Michael Keaton also doesn't really move his lips when he talks. Much of the movie is shot with the characters in shadow, or with their hands in front of their faces. The first rule of speech-reading is that the speaker's lips have to be visible. A no-brainer.

Neil Bauman has written a number of columns about speech-reading on the website Hearing Loss Help.[124] Bauman's column is generally framed in a question-and-answer format, and readers do seem to ask the same questions over and over again: Can you learn speech-reading? How? Are there classes?

You *can* learn to speech-read and there *are* classes, though they are few and far between. Most people with long-term hearing loss, especially from childhood, learn to read lips by experience. A minimal amount of residual hearing is almost a prerequisite, though some people can speech-read with no hearing at all. This means they can speech-read at a distance. An example of this was the professional speech-reader Tina Lannan, who watched the Royal Wedding, featuring William and Kate, and disclosed several private conversations to the media. My favorite was Queen Elizabeth's comment that she wished William and Kate had decided to take the smaller carriage. (Why, one wonders. Modesty? That it was the same carriage Charles and Diana used? That it was looking a little tattered? No clue.)

Successful speech-reading depends on a number of factors, among them the lighting and environmental conditions, the way the speaker articulates, and the way the listener (you) observes.

The Ideal Speech-Reading Environment

The venue has to be well lit, or at least light enough for you to see the speaker's lips. If the speaker is backlit by a window or a bright light, you won't be able to see the face clearly—just a silhouette. The area lighting should be constant, no flickering shadows or blinking lights. Speech-reading under a strobe light would be all but impossible. Don't expect to have a conversation if you go out dancing on New Year's Eve.

You'll understand more in a quiet room where you'll also be able to pick up sound with your residual hearing. But it is possible to train yourself to pick out one voice from among others. Technology helps with this. If the speaker is wearing your FM transmitter, that will help tremendously. My Naida cochlear implant from Advanced Bionics has a "zoom" program that helps me focus on one speaker.

It's difficult to speech-read around a table. Some people find it easier if the table is round, because everyone is facing inward. I still find this difficult, because some speakers will be in profile even at a round table. At a square or rectangular table, you will probably have trouble with people sitting on the same side of the table with you, in full profile.

I belong to a book club made up of eight old friends. I've thought of having them all face me—as if we were in a classroom with me as the teacher, or an interrogation with me on one side of the table and everyone else on the other. Just a fantasy. But I did email everyone in the book club the link to a slide show on speech-reading that I read about in one of Neil Bauman's columns. "I Hear with My Eyes,"[125] by Cynthia Dixon, is both funny and very helpful. My friends appreciated the specific suggestions.

When Speech-Reading Is Difficult

You often hear the remark that someone's expression is unreadable, or that someone is stony faced. Sometimes it's a neutral description—think of Ed Sullivan or Buster Keaton. More often the term is applied to disgruntled heads of state or assassins—the term suggests not just a lack of affect but a negative affect.

The opposite is someone animated, whose facial expression reflects what she is saying. The eyes are especially revealing, and a close observer can read an expression from the eyes (and eyebrows) alone. (Speech-reading a person in dark sunglasses can be difficult.) A speech-reader will have a much easier time understanding someone animated, at least as long as the person is not too animated. As I said in my previous book, shouting won't help, in part because shouting distorts the face.

A beard or mustache almost always obscures the lips. Some people have thin lips, or they don't move their lips when they talk. If you're at a party, you won't be able to speech-read if the speaker is looking over your head or around the room or even down at the floor for some reason. You won't be able to understand someone eating. You won't be able to follow people who flutter their hands in front of their faces. You won't be able to understand someone smoking or chewing gum. You won't be able to understand someone laughing—like shouting, it distorts the mouth.

It is also difficult to speech-read a person with a speech impediment or a foreign accent. I have a hard time following someone who has been deaf from birth and has a strong "deaf accent." This is especially troubling because that person probably already feels sensitive about his speech. I also have a hard time following young children.

One situation where speech-reading failed to help me was when my mother was very old and in a nursing facility. Her voice got whispery, and she'd had a stroke so she didn't enunciate or move her lips much. Her caregivers would try to fill me in, but they had strong South Carolina accents, and I couldn't follow them, either. Frustrating and sometimes heartbreaking.

Also frustrating, but not heartbreaking, is trying to hear my hairdresser as he cuts my hair. I have to take off my hearing aid and implant so they don't get in the way of his scissors. I don't hear much. The salon is full of noisy hair dryers, my hairdresser has a foreign accent, and most important, I'm trying to read his lips in the mirror. Without my glasses. It doesn't seem to bother him.

Train Your Brain

Some people are intuitively good speech-readers, but it is possible to train yourself. It takes practice and it's hard because the way sounds are formed is often not visible. Only about 30 to 40 percent of English sounds can be seen on the speaker's lips. The rest are formed in the throat or in the way the tongue touches the teeth.

You can start by learning to really look at a speaker. Stare at the person, in fact. Body language and facial expression can tell you a lot. So can context.

The journalist (and now mystery writer) Henry Kisor lost his hearing after a bout with meningitis and encephalitis at age three. He has spent his whole life reading lips, and wrote about it in his now classic 1991 memoir called *What's That Pig Outdoors?* The title comes from an anecdote where he misreads his young son's question, "What's that big loud noise?" They look identical on the lips.

So do words like *map*, *bat*, and *pat*. That's because the letters *m*, *b*, and *p* look alike on a speaker's lips. As in Henry Kisor's sentence, *big* and *pig* also look alike. Neil Bauman points out that the words *queen* and *white* look alike on the lips, even though they sound completely different. That's why context is important.

But context doesn't always help. A hearing-impaired man, Mr. A., runs into his old friend Mr. B. Thanks to similar-sounding words, the conversation goes like this: *Mr. A: By the way, how is your brother? Mr. B: My brother was buried last week. Mr. A. Wonderful! You must be very pleased about that.* To someone with hearing loss, "buried" and "married" are homophones. This example comes from *Speechreading: A Way to Improve Understanding*, by Harriet Kaplan, Scott J. Bally, and Carol Garretson.[126] It's a useful and readable discussion of the principles of speech-reading, its limitations, some listening strategies, and practical exercises.

Resources for Practicing

You can improve your speech-reading skills, but speech-reading alone will never replace hearing. Almost everyone needs at least some residual hearing, knowledge of sign language, or the help of hearing assistive technology.

Gallaudet University offers a comprehensive list of speech-reading resources, including books, DVDs, and videotapes, and even a parlor game.[127] The game, "Read My Lips: The Wild Party Game of Unspoken Words," can be ordered from the manufacturer, Pressman Toy Corporation, or on Amazon or eBay.

One of the most helpful resources Gallaudet offers is a pamphlet called "Speechreading in Context: A Guide to Everyday Settings." It can be downloaded for free as a PDF or ordered for $3 (to cover shipping and handling). I came upon this helpful resources page on About.com,[128] which also mentions other publications and allows you to compare book prices.

Speech-reading classes do exist but they can be hard to find. The Gallaudet "Resources" page suggests trying your otolaryngologist, a local hearing and speech center, a state professional association, or a university training hospital. It also recommends contacting the AG Bell Association, HLAA, and other organizations for those with hearing loss.

The Center for Hearing and Communication (CHC) offers speech-reading classes at its Manhattan location (at 50 Broadway) and claims to be New York's only speech-reading program. This may be true, as speech-reading instruction is rare. CHC recommends six to ten individual sessions, to learn the theoretical underpinnings of the way speech is formed in the mouth. After that, a person might decide to attend small-group sessions for practice with others and with an instructor.

Sometimes insurance will cover these classes. After I got my cochlear implant, I took individual auditory rehabilitation classes at CHC with Linda Kessler, who also teaches speech-reading. My insurance (UnitedHealthcare) did not cover the $100 per session, though it did cover other kinds of therapy, including physical therapy (for a non-hearing issue) and psychotherapy.

Google "speech-reading classes" and you'll find reliable and unreliable resources, including classes offered by individuals. You'd probably want to double check with a local hearing center to see if it can vouch for the specific program. Add your location to the Google search bar and you'll find local offerings.

Gael Hannan has given several workshops on teaching speech-reading, including one called "Man-Lips: Men and Speechreading—Facing the Challenge." It turns out there is a gender difference in speech-reading success, or at least it seems that way for those with acquired hearing loss. The perception is that women do it better.

Three factors may contribute, including the way men and women articulate. More persuasive, though, is the fact that men are less comfortable with sustained eye contact than women, and that they are less comfortable showing emotion. Hannan suggests that if you want to run a male-inclusive speech-reading course, promote it as a "success strategy" and incorporate lots of gadgets.

Even the best speech-readers are stymied by certain situations. As Hannan wrote in a 2011 blog post: "What's my worst speech-reading nightmare? A Scotsman, fresh off the boat from the highlands, talking with beer foam on his bushy mustache. No matter how slowly the wee man might speak, I can nae understand a word!"

CHAPTER TWENTY

What the Heck Is a Hearing Loop?

"For the first time since I lost most of my hearing, live music was perfectly clear, perfectly clean and incredibly rich."[129]

There is only one circumstance under which I can begin to understand what's being said without seeing the speaker's lips. That's in a room, even in an auditorium-size room—in fact even in the 12,000-seat Michigan State basketball arena, should I ever find myself there—in which an audio frequency induction loop, popularly known as a hearing loop or just a loop, has been installed.

"Looping" is a technology based on the principle of electromagnetic fields. From the user perspective, it's incredibly simple. You simply sit or stand in the designated area, flip your hearing aid to telecoil mode, and sound—from a lecturer at a podium, from your TV set, from any audio source—should come through loud and clear.

Installing the system is not simple, however. It involves running a wire around the periphery of a room or, in a large auditorium, between rows of seats. The wire runs either under the floor or carpeting or in the ceiling. The microphone in the room picks up the speaker's voice and sends it to the sound system. The sound system sends the audio signal to the loudspeakers, for the normal hearing audience, but also to the loop amplifier. The loop amplifier and wire create a weak magnetic field surrounding the listening area. The telecoil in the listener's hearing aid or cochlear implant picks up the signal and converts it into sound, which seems to go directly from the speaker at the podium (or the TV) into the listener's ear.

Essentially, the speaker's voice is as clear as if he or she were four feet in front of you. Clearer perhaps, because of the elimination of background noise.

Looping involves no extra gadgets on the user's part, as long as the hearing aid or cochlear implant is equipped with a manual telecoil. As I noted earlier, all cochlear implants have telecoils, and so do most hearing aids, though you may have to ask for it or ask to have it activated.

Looping: Then and Now

Looping has been around for a long time. In 1937, Joseph Poliakoff, a Soviet émigré and sound engineer, applied for a British patent on an "Induction Loop Hearing Assistance System." The key to the system was what was then known as a Telephone Coil, which was designed to pick up the audio signal from a telephone handset's magnetic field. The telephone coil transmitted the audio signal to a hearing aid. The first T-coil–enabled hearing aid came on the market in 1938. (The hearing aid consisted of a vest-pocket body pack connected to earphones.)

An induction loop system is a logical extension of the telephone technology. In a looped space, the loop wire basically surrounds the user, picking up signals from the audio amplifier. Looping began to come into widespread use in the 1970s after Britain's National

Health Service began distributing hearing aids fitted with telecoils. The stage was set for a technology that could take advantage of them.

Early systems were hit and miss. The effects of structural metal (in beams, for instance) and dimensions of the loop were not well understood. These early glitches gave looping a bad name in some circles, but it has long had strong proponents. In 2007, the International Electrotechnical Commission (IEC) instituted a new Induction Loop Standard. Newer loop systems adhering to this standard provide a far more consistent magnetic signal. It takes a trained installer to make sure the loop is installed properly. It's not a do-it-yourself project, although there is one exception. A loop "cushion" on your favorite TV chair, linked to a TV loop, costs about $400 and is, according to some experts, "easy to install." (For some of us, nothing technological is easy to install.)

For someone like me, to hear a lecture in a well-looped auditorium is nothing short of miraculous. Unfortunately, I haven't had many opportunities to do that, because so far looping has not caught on widely in the United States. (The United Kingdom, and some European countries, remains way ahead of the United States in the use of looping systems.) Every meeting of the national HLAA or our New York City chapter is held in a space with either permanent or temporary looping. But cultural venues have been slow to pick up the technology.

Two states, Michigan and Wisconsin, are much more widely looped, thanks to the efforts of two individuals: David G. Myers, a psychology professor at Hope College in Holland, Michigan, and Juliette Sterkens, an audiologist from Wisconsin. Myers has hearing loss, as did his mother, and has become a major advocate for hearing loops. His website, HearingLoop.org, provides all sorts of practical information. Myers energized the Let's Loop America campaign, which is now backed by major hearing loss and professional organizations. Sterkens's work raised awareness of the benefits of loops among consumers, ministers, and hearing care professionals in her state, which caused a surge in loop installations. She's a passionate, persuasive speaker, and I'm sure has prompted the installation of many loop systems throughout the country.

In New York City, thanks again to the efforts of a few individuals, a variety of cultural and civic institutions now are looped, including all of New York City's MTA subway booths. (A plan to loop New York City taxis is coming along more slowly.) You can find a list of looped environments at HLAA NYC. Other local chapters of HLAA include information about looping in their areas.

Seattle is another city with a strong loop advocate. Seattle's primary lecture venue, historic Town Hall, is in the process of installing permanent hearing loops in all three of its major spaces, as part of an overall renovation.

I'm so used to relying on captions that sometimes I forget to turn on my telecoil when I'm in a looped environment. This happened to me recently at an HLAA board meeting. I'm the board secretary (thanks to my typing skills). When a recent meeting convened, I got out my laptop to take notes. I found myself relying on the CART screen frequently. It was only at the break that I remembered the room was looped. For the rest of the meeting, I was able to hear and understand almost everything that was said, with only occasional glances at the CART screen to fill in the blanks.

Richard Einhorn, the composer and sound engineer, experienced sudden hearing loss in 2010, a result of otosclerosis. Einhorn was featured in a 2011 article in *The New York Times* about looping, titled "A Hearing Aid That Cuts Out All the Clatter." Einhorn had recently experienced looping for the first time: "There I was at *Wicked* weeping uncontrollably—and I don't even like musicals," he said. "For the first time since I lost most of my hearing, live music was perfectly clear, perfectly clean and incredibly rich."

David Myers had a similar reaction to Richard's, way back in 1999 when he first heard looped sound at Scotland's ancient Iona Abbey. "My wife noticed a hearing assistance sign with a 'T' and nudged me to turn on the 'telecoils' in my new aids. The instant result was a stunningly clear voice, speaking from the center of my head. I was in tears."

My first exposure to looping was less emotional. It was at the 2012 Hearing Loss Association of America conference in Providence, Rhode Island. This was not my first HLAA conference, but it was the first with a telecoil in my hearing aid. The year before I'd frantically followed the CART transcription of that year's fascinating research symposium, on hearing and noise. (The full transcript was published later, which helped fill in many blanks in my hastily typed notes.)

I got there just in time for the keynote address, given by David Myers. I turned on my new telecoils and listened as Myers described a trip to the U.K., the center of the world for induction loops. I not only heard every word but could even detect his Midwestern accent. Dr. Myers described taking the rail transfer into the city, connecting from there to the tube. Both were looped. In visits to the British Library, the Tower of London, Westminster Abbey, he could ask questions and hear the answers. Certain British Rail cars are looped, so he could hear announcements on the train. When he got to Canterbury Cathedral, it, like virtually every house of worship in Britain, was looped. Even the golf course at St. Andrews had looped information kiosks. When he went to send a postcard home, he found the post office information booth was looped.

I went to an international conference on looping in Eastbourne, on the English Channel, a year or so later. The conference hall was looped, and I heard every word. So were many other local venues. One reason the loop worked so well was that it was installed by trained loop installers to the IEC Standard.

But as good as the experience is when it's working, I have often found myself floundering where I expected to hear clear speech. Looping does not always work, unfortunately. In general, the fault lies in imprecise installation or in "user" error (the speaker does not speak into the mic correctly) or because the listener's telecoils were improperly installed.

At an HLAA convention in Austin, Texas, the reception desk in the hotel was looped. I could hear every word said to the man next to me but nothing said to me. Again, this was user error: The mic was not in the proper position.

I was invited to speak at Seattle Town Hall at a celebration of the decision to loop the hall. A temporary loop had been installed (the renovation and permanent installation will begin in 2016). Unfortunately, many of the audience members heard not only my talk but also the talk being given in the auditorium downstairs. Installers got back to work on the temporary loop the next day.

In 2012, the Baltimore Symphony temporarily looped its concert hall, with the collaboration of the Hearing Loss Association of America, for a performance of Richard Einhorn's *Voices of Light*, a symphonic work with a chorus, which accompanies the classic silent film *The Passion of Joan of Arc*. When I asked Einhorn what it was like to hear his music again, expecting a rhapsodic response similar to the thrill he'd felt at *Wicked*, he said the loop system hadn't been working properly where he sat.

Looping is still in its infancy—or, at least, early childhood—and the technology is challenging. But where loops are installed properly and the microphone inputs from the PA systems are integrated as they should be, it's terrific. Like many in the hearing loss field, I have high hopes for it.

Surprisingly, people without hearing problems who have tried a hearing loop (using headphones), report that they, too, hear much more clearly through the loop.

A study at Northern Illinois University's Audiology Clinic[130] included hearing and non-hearing participants. Testing was done in a reverberant auditorium and included hearing-in-noise tests as well as others; 99 percent of the participants reported they could hear better with the hearing loop (the hearing participants wore headphones with a telecoil). The surprise was that 48 percent of the *hearing* subjects were so impressed by these improvements, they said they would use a telecoil in a looped environment.

Think of the Possibilities

nduction loops have all sorts of possibilities. Here are some that are probably not ever going to happen (no reason not to indulge in some wishful thinking), some that might happen, and some that may be happening already.

A concert where every musician and singer was wearing a mic, so that it would all come clearly right into my head.[131]

A child who is deaf or hard of hearing gets along in mainstream classrooms because the teacher wears a transmitter and the student wears an FM receiver. But if another student says something—and is not wearing a mic—the deaf student can't hear it. This is an issue that has been addressed in a few venues by voice-activated mics on cords hanging from the ceiling or by passing around a hand mic. But again, the distance from the speaker would result in an imperfect signal. Tiny mics for each student, which would cut out when more than one student spoke at a time, would be amazing! One of the issues for deaf and hard of hearing children is not being able to hear other students, which can impact the value of their education.

Looping in a restaurant, again with each speaker miked. This is currently not possible because the loops would bleed into each other because of the closeness of the tables in a restaurant.

My dinner table at Thanksgiving. Eighteen people each wearing a mic. Of course they all talk at once, so maybe I, the listener, could have a control to focus on whatever person I thought might be saying the most interesting thing.

And, of course, if it got too noisy, I could just turn the whole thing off. Hearing loss has its benefits.

CHAPTER TWENTY-ONE

Cochlear Implants

Where once I was deaf, now I hear.

Chances are your hearing loss will worsen as the years go by. If the loss is noise-related, continued exposure to noise as well as the natural deterioration in hearing that comes with aging will take their toll. If you have hearing loss from some other cause, it may well be progressive.

Even if you are assiduously using the assistive listening devices discussed in Chapter 18, like an FM system to boost the performance of your hearing aid, or have access to an induction loop at a house of worship or a lecture hall, or even in your own living room, you may eventually find you're missing a lot. The phone becomes harder to use; speech becomes difficult to understand even in minimally noisy environments. That's partly because hearing aids, even the best, primarily amplify rather than clarify. You hear someone speaking but can't understand what he or she is saying.

These can be indications that you might be a candidate for a cochlear implant.

How They Work

Cochlear implants are one of the great medical advances of the twentieth century, and in 2014 three researchers were awarded the Lasker Prize, often referred to as America's Nobel, for their role in developing the technology.

Hearing aids amplify sounds and send them through the ear canal to the inner ear, where they are picked up by the remaining undamaged hair cells. When all the cells are damaged or destroyed, you might need a cochlear implant. Cochlear implants bypass the outer and middle ear and deliver electronic signals directly to the auditory nerve.

A cochlear implant consists of several connected components, some external and some implanted in the skull. The external components are the software, and are upgraded every three to five years. The earpiece, located behind the ear, consists of a microphone to capture the sound, a speech processor that transforms the sound into electrical signals, and a rechargeable battery (some come with disposable batteries). Connected to the earpiece by a two-inch cable is the transmitter, a magnetized disk about the size of a quarter. The transmitter attaches magnetically to the implanted receiver, which decodes the signals and sends them through an internal cable into the cochlea. At the end of the cable are a series of electrodes (the number of electrodes differs according to brand), which snake into the spiral interior of the cochlea, lining up with receptors on the auditory nerve, bypassing the severely damaged or destroyed hair cells. The auditory nerve relays the information to the brain, which translates the signals into recognizable sounds.

The implant works only when the external magnetized transmitter is attached. The user takes the earpiece and transmitter off at night, for comfort, or when swimming or engaged in other activities that might damage it. (New waterproof designs allow some models to be kept on while in the water.) Without the earpiece and transmitter sending it signals, the implanted receiver is inactive. Unless you rub your hand over that part of your skull, you could even forget you had it. The implant feels like a quarter-size plateau above and behind your ear.

Cochlear implants are not for everyone. If you can hear with a hearing aid fairly well, you'll do better to stick with the hearing aid than to get a cochlear implant. As of 2013, roughly 58,000 adults and 38,000 children had received implants in the United States. Approximately 324,200 people worldwide have them.

A decade ago, implants were largely restricted to those with profound hearing loss in both ears, but they are now an option for people with some residual hearing. Today they are sometimes recommended for people who are deaf in one ear if they have moderate to severe hearing loss in the other. The cutoff point for the good ear is the ability to recognize no more than 40–50 percent of the words on a word test. (The percentage varies according to manufacturer and insurance carrier.)

In Europe, cochlear implants are used even if the hearing in the good ear is normal, especially if the individual has tinnitus in the bad ear. Darius Kohan, who performed my 2009 implant surgery, told me that American surgeons are starting to implant these patients. They've had great success in minimizing tinnitus, which can be very difficult to treat, and restoring some audition in the poor hearing ear.

Also until recently, the cochlear implant was useful only for those with damage to the hair cells in the inner ear. Newer cochlear implants work with other kinds of hearing loss, and I'll discuss them at the end of this chapter.

Getting a Cochlear Implant

The first step in getting a cochlear implant is to find a surgeon. My longtime ear doctor, Ronald Hoffman at New York Eye and Ear Infirmary (NYEE), was an accomplished and experienced cochlear implant surgeon. In fact, he was part of the team that did the first multichannel implant on a child, in 1986. But he wasn't in my health plan, and rather than run the risk of delays or even a refusal from my insurance company, I chose a surgeon who was in my plan and was recommended by Dr. Hoffman.

I had met Darius Kohan that summer, when Dr. Hoffman referred me to him as a last-ditch effort to reverse or improve my now profound left ear loss. The procedure involved injecting steroids directly into my eardrum, which was just as unpleasant as it sounds. After we did two sessions of the scheduled three and nothing had changed, Dr. Kohan suggested we stop torturing me and move ahead with the plans for the cochlear implant.

His office made all the arrangements for insurance coverage and helped set up the appointments necessary before surgery, including a CT scan to make sure there was nothing that would interfere with placing the implant. Dr. Kohan did surgery at NYEE only a day or two per week, so his schedule was limited. The soonest date available was September 11. Like many New Yorkers, I'm superstitious about that date, but after the 11th he wasn't available for another month, so we went ahead with it.

Both Dr. Hoffman and Dr. Kohan thought I was an ideal candidate for an implant. I had almost profound hearing loss in one ear and partial hearing in the other, and I was motivated. But it's not always such an open-and-shut case. Even if you qualify for a cochlear implant, there are good reasons not to get one, or to wait. Your doctor or audiologist may feel that your particular loss won't benefit from an implant. Or the doctor might suggest you wait for improved technology. Sometimes the patient doesn't want surgery, or doesn't want an implant for other reasons. The metallic receiver implanted in the skull used to preclude an MRI, although under emergencies it can be surgically removed. Med-El has already received FDA approval for an implant that can be left in during the most common kinds of scans (the 1.5 Tesla MRI scans) and both Cochlear and Advanced Bionics are expected to come out with them soon.

If you decide to pursue the cochlear implant option, your audiologist or doctor may suggest implant centers or surgeons in your area. Dr. Neil Bauman on Hearing Loss Help has some practical suggestions about finding a good implant surgeon.[132] Basically, it's a matter of word of mouth, knowing whose recommendation to trust, and doing some Web research. You definitely want a center that does a lot of implants, and you want to make sure it has audiologists and speech-language pathologists on staff.

Make sure you feel comfortable with the audiologist, because she will be your main contact after the surgery. Finally, think about how hard it will be to get to the implant center. You'll need to visit it several times a month initially, so you don't want it to be too distant.

Cochlear implant surgery is getting more routine every day. Nevertheless, you don't want a surgeon who's inexperienced. The surgery is delicate, with the incision running close to the facial nerve. To qualify to perform cochlear implant surgery, an otolaryngologist must not only be a specialist in head and neck surgery but must be specifically trained in otology/neurotology, a two-year training program and a second board certification. At one point, implant surgery was associated with meningitis, so most implant centers require a meningitis vaccine. But as the incisions get smaller, meningitis is rarely, if ever, a problem.

The surgeon has probably recommended your worse ear for the implant, which means that you may still have some normal hearing (possibly with a hearing aid) in the good ear. The idea is to preserve as much hearing as possible in the "good" ear, both because natural hearing, even with a hearing aid, is a benefit and because it wouldn't make sense to take a chance with the good ear. Since the cochlear implant destroys the hair cells in the process of insertion, you'd be wiping out your valuable residual hearing.

If you are deaf in both ears, you would benefit from bilateral implants. But many public and private insurers in the United States will cover only one, if that. National Health in the U.K. will pay for one cochlear implant. In a case like mine, aging into Medicare can be beneficial. My private insurance company paid for my first implant, in 2009. I expect that Medicare will pay for a second in my other ear, though this is not a given. (Medicare did, however, pay for the five-year upgrade of my external processor.) If you do get two cochlear implants, your surgeon may suggest doing them one at a time, not to ease the experience for you but to make sure that the first one works before inserting the second. Very rarely (in about 1.5 percent of cases) the internal component of an implant may fail. Replacing this would require a second surgery.

Although the surgery requires a skilled surgeon, it's relatively easy for the patient. Done on an outpatient basis, it takes between one and two hours. Infants as young as six or eight months old are implanted, as are adults into their nineties. The internal device is permanent. It doesn't need to be replaced as a child grows, though the external elements will be upgraded at intervals.

The surgery is much less invasive than, say, anything involving the cardiovascular system or a hip or knee replacement, and it requires a much briefer recovery period than most surgical procedures. I was up and walking across the park to a follow-up appointment with Dr. Kohan three days after the surgery. You will have a raw wound behind the ear for a week or two, and in the days immediately following surgery, your head will be swathed in a kind of gauze turban. It reminded me of the headgear in *Swan Lake*. Most implant centers wait a month for full healing before the implant is activated.

Activation takes place in the audiologist's office, and it's a big moment. Even though the connections were tested during surgery, there's still no way to guarantee that the implant will work. For someone deaf since early childhood or birth, the very existence of sound in the ear can be a breathtaking experience. It can also be a jarring experience, though, for anyone. The sound initially may be harsh and unarticulated.

The audiologist gets to work programming the device, based on your feedback. By the time you leave the office, you may be able to understand some speech and begin to recognize some sounds. You'll want to keep the implant on all the time and begin practicing with it right from the start. (For more about auditory rehabilitation, see "Train Your Brain" later in this chapter.) Your audiologist may recommend that you not wear your hearing aid for the first few weeks, to help with acclimating your brain to the sounds produced by the cochlear implant.

Choosing Brands

Some surgeons have brand preferences, but most say the three major brands are equally effective. The number of electrodes in the three varies, as does the technology, but this doesn't affect how well recipients will hear. A few months before I got my cochlear implant, Dr. Kohan handed me three packets of information from the three implant companies with FDA approval: MED-EL, Cochlear, and Advanced Bionics. These same brands are the ones used in the U.K., which also adds the Digisonic from Neurelec, a French company now owned by Oticon Medical.

I was at a loss, and reading online comments from users of the various brands wasn't much help. You get only one chance at an implant: You can't trade it in for a different model (without enormous expense and a second surgery), so most people naturally—and hopefully—assume they made the right choice. There are some people who have different brands in different ears, but that's complicated for a lot of reasons.

I came upon a valuable article about the various brands recently, which appeared on the blog "I Look So I Can Hear."[133] It discusses the pluses and minuses of specific brands in detail. The comments are also interesting, and not always in agreement with the original article or with other comments. The variety of opinions allows readers to make their own judgments.

One thing I didn't do, and wish I had, was try on the earpieces of the three manufacturers. At the time, the earpiece of the Advanced Bionics Harmony model, which I ended up getting, was larger than some of the others, and I had a hard time keeping it on behind my ear. Advanced Bionics now has a sleeker model, the Naida, and I was eligible to upgrade to the new earpiece in September 2014, five years after I got my first implant. It's slightly narrower and it still tends to slip off my ear, but a plastic clip is available and I often wear the earpiece clipped to my shirt or my hair instead of behind my ear.

Using the clip means I have a visible wire running to the magnet on my head. In these days of devices in everyone's ears—from iPods to Bluetooth and onward—a wire isn't a big deal. But the clip itself is ugly and even uglier with the cochlear implant attached. Someone can make a lot of money by designing an attractive cover for the clip, which might look like a colorful pin or disk.

Cochlear implant companies tend to play hopscotch with features—one offers a waterproof implant and then so do the others. Some claim to be better at hearing music. Some offer behind-the-ear processors in vibrant colors and some are plain vanilla. (My favorite was a black earpiece studded with rhinestones, which I saw on a woman at one of the HLAA conventions.) Some claim longer battery life (the batteries are rechargeable). Other considerations are the weight of the batteries and charger, especially if you travel a lot.

You might want a waterproof model if you're a swimmer or athlete. It's also good to look at performance history to see if there have been recent recalls or other issues.

Other Kinds of Cochlear Implants

In early 2014, the FDA approved an implant that preserves residual hearing, an important advance. The tail with the electrode array is shorter, meaning it goes less deeply into the spiral of the cochlea. The hair cells that aren't affected, in the lower frequencies, aren't damaged. Many people with the most common kinds of hearing loss, the result of noise or age damage, have hearing problems in the high frequencies but hear well enough in the low. These hybrids combine cochlear implant technology for the high frequencies with hearing aid technology (essentially, amplification) for the low frequencies.

Cochlear Corporation's Nucleus Hybrid L24 was the first of these shorter devices to be approved in the United States, in March 2014. MED-EL and Advanced Bionics are close behind. The FDA's news release[134] about the Cochlear Hybrid L24 discussed both the benefits and some possible "adverse events," including low frequency hearing loss, tinnitus, and dizziness. But, it concluded, "While the risk of low frequency hearing loss is of concern, the FDA determined that the overall benefits of the device outweigh this risk for those who do not benefit from traditional hearing aids. Prospective patients should carefully discuss all benefits and risks of this new device with their physicians. The device is intended for use on one ear only."

Some people can't use hearing aids because their deafness is the result of incomplete development of the outer or middle ear or chronic infection in the ear. But they may have a fully functional cochlea. Most surgeons would be reluctant to use a conventional cochlear implant in this situation, because it destroys the hair cells.

For these people, the solution is an implant that conducts sound through bone. Cochlear's bone-anchored cochlear implant, the

Baha,[135] was approved in 2002, making it the most venerable. The Ponto, and Ponto Pro,[136] made by Oticon Medical, and the Alpha 1 Hearing System by Sophono, Inc. also now have FDA approval.[137]

The audio processor, which is held in place directly above the implant by magnetic attraction, records the sound and converts it into signals, which are then transferred through the skin to the implant. The implant is embedded in the temporal bone and converts the signals received into mechanical vibrations that are then transmitted to the surrounding bone.

The bone then conducts these vibrations to the inner ear where they are converted into nerve signals and transmitted as impulses to the auditory nerve, similar to the natural hearing process.[138]

In previous versions of the Baha, the abutment penetrated the skin of the skull. Now the magnet is often underneath the skin, like a conventional cochlear implant. In December 2013, Cochlear introduced the Baha 4 Attract, which connects magnetically to the implanted device, eliminating the need for the skin-penetrating abutment.[139] The vibrations are transmitted through the bony shell of the cochlea and, via the cochlear fluid, stimulate the auditory nerve to carry signals to the brain.

The Baha was originally designed for single-sided hearing, when there is no hearing in one ear and normal hearing in the other. The vibration is passed through the skull to the hearing ear. Like conventional implants, the Baha has a telecoil, which can be used with various wireless assistive listening devices. The Baha is not recommended for children under five. For these children, Cochlear Ltd. makes the Baha Softband, which looks like a colorful headband and is removable. (Adults who don't want surgery can also use this method.)

In June of 2014, the Centers for Medicare and Medicaid Services (CMS) proposed to reclassify bone-anchored implants as hearing aids, which would mean they were no longer covered under Medicare. While noting that the savings would not be significant, the CMS inexplicably decided this was a good decision anyway.[140]

Surprisingly, and in a triumph for the power of advocacy, CMS reversed the decision several months later.

Paying for Your Cochlear Implant

Most private insurers as well as Medicare, Medicaid, and the VA will pay for a cochlear implant if you meet the minimum criteria, as will the NHS in the U.K. As I said earlier, that means a profound loss in the bad ear and a moderate to profound hearing loss in your better ear, with word recognition under 40–50 percent. The cochlear implant center generally takes responsibility for obtaining prior authorization for the implant surgery and also helps set up pre-implant tests, like a CT scan to make sure there is no structural abnormality that would rule out a cochlear implant.

Getting insurance approval is essential because the surgery, the device itself, and the post-surgical care can come to anywhere between $40,000 and $70,000, and maybe even more in some areas. This covers the surgery, the device, and pre- and post-implantation care by the surgeon and by an audiologist.

Hearing with a Cochlear Implant

The rule of thumb for adults is that the sooner you have the implant after losing your hearing, the better you will do with it. That being said, success with an implant is not a given, and it's not predictable.

The first cochlear implant to be approved by the FDA, in 1984, was a single-channel device that allowed users to hear sirens or other loud noises but not to discriminate speech. Today cochlear implants are multichannel, and many people do very well with them. Many people with cochlear implants still need to supplement their implant with lip-reading, assistive devices like captioned telephones, and FM systems. Many cannot hear speech in noise.

We hear with our brains, and nowhere is this more apparent than with cochlear implants. A cochlear implant does not restore normal hearing but rather sends information to the brain, where it gets interpreted as language. How accurately the brain processes these signals varies from person to person. David B. Pisoni at the Indiana University School of Medicine has written a number of academic papers on speech perception after cochlear implantation.[141] In an email to me, Dr. Pisoni explained that each person's brain "adjusts, adapts and codes and processes" these signals differently. To make matters more complicated, the signals from a cochlear implant are, in his terms, "incomplete" or "highly degraded" compared to those that reach the brain of a hearing person.

People who do well with their cochlear implants (over time, and usually after some form of auditory rehabilitation) are, again in Pisoni's words, able to learn to "rapidly encode, store, and process highly degraded, compromised, and underspecified speech signals from their CI." In other words, it's not the signal itself that determines success but the way the user's brain processes it.

That doesn't mean that cochlear implants themselves don't need improving. We've come a long way from the one-channel original, but for many people understanding speech except under ideal circumstances—and for almost everyone, hearing music—remains challenging. Researchers are taking various approaches to this issue. Some are working with the hardware, some are experimenting with novel ways of programming implants, the implant companies themselves are always tinkering with the technology. Researchers are also studying the potential benefits of pairing a cochlear implant in one ear with either another cochlear implant or a hearing aid in the other ear, using wireless technology.

Train Your Brain

The most important factor in learning to hear with a cochlear implant is teaching the brain to recognize these strange new signals as words and recognizable sounds.

This is done through auditory rehabilitation. Working with a speech-language pathologist or an audiologist is mandated for children receiving implants; in their case it's more accurately referred to as auditory habilitation, no "re-," because they're learning to hear for the first time.

Cochlear implant centers differ in their attitudes toward rehab for adults. At the Cochlear Implant Center at the New York Eye and Ear Infirmary, where I got my implant, formal rehab is offered on an "as needed" basis. (The center has a large speech-language pathology team but it works mostly with children, which is mandated by state law.) NYEE generally suggests that patients use the at-home rehab programs offered by the manufacturer of their implant, or online programs like the LACE program.[142]

The website for Cochlear Americas includes an excellent article, "Cochlear Implant Rehabilitation: It's Not Just for Kids!" that's full of information on all aspects of auditory therapy.[143]

Angel Sound is a PC-based interactive listening rehabilitation program developed by TigerSpeech. Advanced Bionics offers The Listening Room[144] on its website, with programs for children, teenagers, and adults. MED-EL's online program is Hear at Home.[145] Each of the companies also has more targeted programs, for instance for talking on the telephone or listening to music.

I turned out to be someone who did need formal auditory rehabilitation, and I was accepted for two twelve-week sessions (a year apart) working with one of NYEE's speech-language pathologists. It helped, though in the end I think what really helped was simply persisting with the cochlear implant, wearing it every waking moment, asking people to repeat things when I didn't understand them, and making an effort to identify every stray sound that I didn't recognize. I still don't do well on word tests with my implant, but combined with my hearing aid it enhances speech perception, and it also gives me a sense of sound location (though not a very good one).

Some centers feel formal rehabilitation is essential. Johns Hopkins, the University of Indiana Medical School, Swedish Hospital in Seattle, the House Institute in L.A., and NYU build rehabilitation into the implant process, just as programming the implant at intervals after the surgery is also part of the package.

Essentially rehab is a way to train your brain to recognize the signals coming from the cochlear implant as specific sounds: being able to distinguish the sound of someone banging the lid on a metal trash can from the sharp bark of a dog or a human shout. They really do all sound alike to the untrained brain. But most important is speech, and rehab focuses on regaining the ability to hear speech clearly, ideally even speech in noise.

The Future of Implant Devices

News about new and improved cochlear implants comes fast and frequently. All three FDA-approved implant manufacturers are coming out with sleeker, more versatile processors and more sophisticated internal devices. Competitors from China (Hangzhou Nurotron Biotechnology.) and France (Neurelec, now owned by Oticon Medical) are pounding on the door.[146]

New devices are being developed all the time. Some aren't exactly hearing aids or cochlear implants. Some also come and go quickly. One that did was Sonitus Medical's SoundBite[147] hearing system, which consisted of a tooth-anchored removable device that transmitted sound from a hearing ear via the teeth to the deaf ear. The CMS, in the decision to leave bone-anchored implants a Medicare-covered device, did not do the same for the SoundBite, classifying it as a hearing aid. The company went out of business.

Auditory Brain Stem Implants (ABIs) can help people with auditory complications—usually a damaged auditory nerve—that make it impossible for them to benefit from a cochlear implant. The electrodes on the ABI stimulate not the auditory nerve but an area of the brain stem known as the cochlear nucleus. Success with speech recognition is mixed, and may be related to the causes of the nerve damage, but some patients have recently achieved speech recognition on a par with cochlear implants. A two-year-old boy was the first child in the United States to receive an ABI, in 2014.[148]

Another innovation, not yet on the market, is the totally implantable cochlear implant. It has no external components and is wirelessly charged using a cell phone. In February 2014, MIT researchers, working with scientists from Harvard Medical School and the Massachusetts Eye and Ear Infirmary, announced that they had developed a new low-powered signal-processing chip that could be used to make a cochlear implant with no external hardware. No clunky earpiece, no wire connecting to the magnetized disk that attaches to the internal receiver.

The device would use the model of a middle-ear hearing aid implant but instead of the sensor detecting the vibrations of the ossicles and mechanically helping the stapes propel sound into the inner ear, the sensor would generate an electrical signal and pass it on to an electrode in the cochlea. The key to this technology is a signal-generating circuit that allows for a chip that uses less power. The chip is recharged wirelessly, either using a phone with an adapter or what the researchers refer to as a "smart pillow." The power would last for about eight hours, at least with current technology. You can read about it in MIT's announcement[149] or in this article in *Physics World*.[150]

Other researchers are working on ways to program existing conventional cochlear implants to improve speech discrimination. The ability to hear music has also become a priority, as the initial goal of providing speech recognition is increasingly achieved.

For now, cochlear implants are not the solution for anyone who can benefit from hearing aids. But as the technology improves, as the costs of the device and the surgery come down, as newer methods of programming and mapping improve the performance of cochlear implants, they may well begin to be seen as an alternative to hearing aids.

News about cochlear implants is outdated almost as soon as it happens. For the most up-to-date information on cochlear implants, keep an eye on the helpful website Cochlear Implant online.[151] The HLAA's website[152] provides a good overview of the issues surrounding cochlear implants, and the FDA's cochlear implant page[153] answers many questions you may have about them. For a good technical explanation of how cochlear implants work, the National Institute on Deafness and Other Communication Disorders (NIDCD) offers a clear and brief summary in this Fact Sheet on Cochlear Implants,[154] which includes illustrations. Johns Hopkins University Medical Center[155] provides a clear description of the implant process for its patients. John Niparko's *Cochlear Implants: Principles and Practices* is the standard reference book for everything having to do with cochlear implants.

PART FIVE

Changing the Way We Think About Hearing Loss

CHAPTER TWENTY-TWO

The Dangers of Denial and Ignorance

Why aren't we wearing hearing aids?

The facts are staggering:

Forty-eight million people in America have hearing loss. The majority are still in the workforce or in school. Ninety percent, or 43.2 million, could benefit from hearing aids.[156] Only 14 percent, or one in seven, have them, and many who have them don't use them with any consistency.

The average age of first-time hearing aid users is approximately seventy,[157] even though half of them began to lose their hearing at least a decade earlier.

This is a lot of people with less than optimal hearing. In most cases it is a hearing loss that could be helped with hearing aids.

If it's that simple, why aren't people wearing them?

Some people with hearing loss think they hear—and under-stand—perfectly well, and they don't *need* to hear better. Others assume that the loss is part of aging and that it would be vanity to try to reverse it, akin to plastic surgery or coloring your hair. Some people with hearing loss either have other, seemingly more impor-tant things to spend their money on or simply can't afford hearing aids. Some are curmudgeons and don't much like hearing other peo-ple anyway, or they're young and think that if they wear hearing aids they'll seem old. Those in the workplace worry that wearing hearing aids will make them look compromised, imperfect, not team players.

While these people are concerned about money and appear-ances, their hearing loss is not only getting worse, it's also becoming a hazard to other aspects of their life and health.

The Dangers of Untreated Hearing Loss

Some people know they have hearing loss and think someday they will get hearing aids—when they need them. There are two prob-lems with this line of thinking.

The first is that they *don't* get them when they need them. In a 1999 National Council on Aging survey, 69 percent of those with hearing loss said the loss wasn't bad enough to require a hearing aid. Nine out of ten of those with mild hearing loss didn't have hear-ing aids. But, worse, six out of ten of those with moderate to severe hearing loss didn't have hearing aids, either.

James Firman, the current head of the National Council on Aging, has moderate to severe hearing loss and wears hearing aids. "I can guarantee you," he said of the responses to this survey, "that there is no way that you are doing fine and getting along fine if that hearing loss is not treated."

One in five respondents said wearing hearing aids would be embarrassing. More embarrassing than seeming stupid or dotty?

"They're not too embarrassed to respond inappropriately, to withdraw from situations, or to be viewed as senile," Firman noted.

The second problem with not getting hearing aids is that untreated hearing loss has physical and psychological consequences that far outweigh the simple inability to hear well. In a series of studies over the years, hearing loss has been linked to depression and social isolation, to paranoia, and to personality changes like becoming more introverted.

But wouldn't poor health in general be associated with social isolation? One study interestingly noted that this is not the case. People in declining overall health, including decreasing ability to function, were no less inclined to socialize, to share experiences, or to express a general sense of well-being. Social withdrawal was specific to hearing loss.

Hearing loss has also been linked to a greater risk of falling. Data from the National Health and Nutrition Examination Survey, which has been gathering information on adults since 1971, show a three-fold increase in the risk of falls among people with a very mild hearing loss (at just 25 dBs). The chances of falling increased with increasing hearing loss.

Several explanations are possible for this. One is that people with poor hearing have a less acute awareness of their environment, making them more prone to tripping. Researcher Frank Lin's cognitive load theory suggests that the brain is distracted by the effort to hear and is "overwhelmed with demands on its limited resources." This sounds a little like saying that walking and chewing gum at the same time results in a cognitive strain. But in fact, Lin says, even though gait and balance are something we take for granted, "they are actually very cognitively demanding. If hearing loss imposes a cognitive load, there may be fewer cognitive resources to help with maintaining balance and gait."

Further, hearing and balance are both controlled by the vestibular system. Hearing loss and balance may be affected by a common cause, like Ménière's. Patients who wore hearing aids performed better on standard balance tests when the aids were turned on than when they were turned off, a study at Washington University School of Medicine found. Timothy M. Hullar, the senior author of the 2014 paper, noted that the patients "appeared to be using the sound information coming through their hearing aids as auditory reference points." He compared the role of hearing in balance to that of vision. "If we turn out the lights, people sway a little bit more."[158]

If you've ever tried to stand on one leg with your eyes closed, you probably know how difficult it is to keep your balance. The senses work in tandem.

Dementia

I've mentioned the correlation between hearing loss and dementia, but I have not discussed the degree to which they are linked, and the ways they negatively affect each other. In a fascinating 2013 paper, M. Kathleen Pichora-Fuller, a psychologist at the University of Toronto, working with colleagues from Toronto, Sweden, and Switzerland, posed a challenge to audiologists and clinicians who work with the elderly.

Their thesis: Treating hearing loss in those with dementia will help to optimize communication, with positive effects on everyday well-being for the patient and the caregivers. Further, treating hearing loss at an earlier stage of cognitive decline may help slow or stave off more severe cognitive loss.

How might this happen? We don't know the underlying explanation for the correlation between hearing loss and dementia, but we do know the correlation exists. Clinical research has shown that hearing loss is found in nine out of ten subjects with dementia. This could be because those with hearing loss are more likely to isolate themselves, which is itself a risk factor for faster cognitive decline.[159]

It could also be that the changes in brain structure that we know accompany hearing loss also affect cognition. Pichora-Fuller encouraged further research into hearing rehabilitation—including but not limited to hearing aids—as a means of offsetting or slowing down the development of dementia.

But most strikingly, as Pichora-Fuller stated, research shows that low scores on speech-in-noise and pure-tone tests are associated with a higher risk of dementia. In other words, you don't have to be deaf to be at higher risk of dementia. All those people who can't hear in restaurants or other noisy places, whose wives mumble, who can't hear on the telephone because the connection is bad—all those people who say they don't need hearing aids—are putting themselves at greater risk for cognitive decline.

What Pichora-Fuller and others are asking is critically important: If we could treat hearing loss at an early stage—when the inability to detect speech in noise is detected, for instance—could we help prevent the change in brain structure that accompanies hearing loss?

In other words, could you fool your brain into thinking you're still a hearing person?—because you are actually, even though technology plays a role.

If we can keep those areas of the brain actively engaged in hearing, are we also keeping them actively involved in the kinds of cognitive activity that may help keep dementia at bay?

Hearing health professionals have long argued that the optimum time for fitting hearing aids is when the older adult is still young enough to be motivated to use them, as well as physically and cognitively able to learn how to use them and how to adjust to the technology. Pichora-Fuller points out that given that average age of first-time hearing aid users (seventy), one in five will likely have a significant cognitive loss by the time they're trying to learn to adapt to hearing aids.

Finally, difficulties in language and cognition are common to both hearing loss and cognitive decline. Correcting the hearing can lead to better cognitive communication.

In March 2015, a French researcher, Isabelle Mosnier, of Assistance Publique-Hopitaux de Paris, published a study on the effect of cochlear implants on elderly patients with hearing loss.[160] Her study was significant not only because she focused on cochlear implants but also because it found not simply a stabilizing effect but improvement in cognition among the most seriously cognitively impaired in the group. One researcher, P. Murali Doraiswamy, M.D., a professor of psychiatry and medicine at Duke University and coauthor of *The Alzheimer's Action Plan*, says that although the study had some shortcomings, "the improvement in cognition was huge (about double that seen with any of the current FDA drugs for treating Alzheimer's)." The patients ranged in age from sixty-five to eighty-five.

The correction doesn't have to be a hearing aid or cochlear implant. Many older people will have trouble with the small size, battery door, and controls. For these, an assistive listening device might be what they need. A PSAP would allow them to interact with caregivers and visitors. An amplified telephone might allow them to keep up with family and friends. Alerting devices could help them be less confused at home about whether the ringing is the telephone or the doorbell, the timer or the alarm clock. FM systems can be used for group activities. TV ears can let them keep up with the news and their favorite TV shows.

Nobody is too old to benefit from hearing help. The brain is never too rigid to change.

The Social Costs of Untreated Hearing Loss

Untreated hearing loss has repercussions far beyond the individual. It results in soaring public-health expenditures, but our silo mentality about health costs obscures that fact. In the United States, our shortsighted view in not underwriting the cost of hearing aids results in billions of dollars spent down the line for treating the consequences of that failure.

In the workplace, untreated hearing loss contributes to underperformance and unemployment. More than half of all people with hearing loss are under the age of sixty, the prime working years, and they are the least likely age group to get hearing aids. The workforce also includes many older people, and as the population ages, so does the number of people with hearing loss. Early retirement, disability retirement, a less productive workforce are all costly.

This is a global problem, and although I've focused on the United States in this book, the issues we face in our wealthy country are exponentially greater in the poor nations of the world. Consider dementia. The World Health Organization projects that the worldwide incidence of dementia will nearly double from 35.6 million in 2010 to 65.7 million in 2030. By 2050, it will triple to 115.4 million people. Seventy percent of this dementia will be in low- and middle-income countries. Treating dementia today costs $600 billion a year. The 2050 cost is estimated at $1.2 trillion (in today's dollars).

In the United States, Frank Lin calculates that by the year 2050, one in thirty Americans will have dementia. He points out that if we could delay the onset of dementia by even one year, its prevalence drops 15 percent down the road.

CHAPTER TWENTY-THREE

What We Can Do

Dispelling the stigma of hearing loss.

The more of us who are open and outspoken about our hearing loss and our need for affordable, effective, and accessible hearing help, the more the market will change to meet that demand. Hearing aid companies are already getting the message, and feeling the competition from the manufacturers of other hearing devices. So are audiologists. Big-box stores like Costco offer full audiological services and hearing aids at half the price, or even less, of elsewhere.

We can defeat the stigma. The more we talk about hearing loss, the more we normalize it. And it is normal: Most people with hearing loss begin to develop it by the age of sixty. By the time we reach our eighties, 90 percent of us have hearing problems. It's time hearing loss is accommodated as routinely as other disabilities.

Our society needs to understand that hearing loss is no different from being nearsighted or having high cholesterol or high blood pressure, or sensitive skin, or allergies. We wouldn't think of ignoring those, and if we did it could be at our peril. Continue with the high-fat diet, don't exercise, and refuse to take a statin and you may end up with a heart attack. Refuse to wear glasses and you trip over things. Fail to use sunscreen and you may end up with melanoma. Continue to ignore your hearing loss and put yourself at risk for falls and dementia.

So what can we do?

We Need a New Model of Hearing Health Care

People don't buy hearing aids, in part because they don't know where to begin. I've given some guidelines in this book. But while most people are vaguely aware that hearing aids might help them, the questions concerning going about getting one are large and amorphous:

What kind of hearing aid do I need? Where should I buy it? How can I afford it? Do I need an audiologist? How do I find one? Hearing aids are not only expensive, but they come in a dizzying array of choices with very little solid evidence to weigh their relative merits.

The growing influence of the big-box stores like Costco may make the decision to buy a hearing aid easier. You're in the store anyway. You see the hearing aid department. You go over for a look. You try one out. Hey, you think, maybe this is a good idea. If it doesn't work out, the cost will be refunded.

Many audiologists, however, *don't* think this is a good idea. They don't want you buying your hearing aid at Costco. But when you ask why, they say the "service" is better at a private audiology clinic. That's not enough: They need to tell us why the service is better. For noise- or age-related hearing loss—that is, everyday hearing loss—the big-box stores seem like a good solution. More than good—because if they get more people wearing hearing aids, we'll all be the better for it. With close to 90 percent of those who could benefit from a hearing aid not using them, shouldn't our goal be getting more hearing help for more people? Getting more help for more people means making hearing aids more accessible and more affordable. And that means selling them in the places that people shop.

We need audiologists to be on board with new approaches and new technologies, especially in cases when a hearing aid isn't enough. As Cynthia Compton-Conley said, we need a new model of hearing care, one where hearing aids are part of a larger package of technologies. As you navigate the world of assistive listening devices, an audiologist will be a crucial guide. That is, an audiologist who is willing to give you time: The time the audiologist needs to assess your specific hearing requirements. And the time you need to ask questions. The audiologist might suggest you buy a cheaper hearing aid if you also get an FM streamer to work with your phone. Or maybe you would benefit from a more expensive hearing aid, plus the Roger Pen. Maybe the audiologist could offer the two together at a discount. Some audiologists do this already. It's not a new idea. But it's rare. With cochlear implants, it's the standard sales model.

Many of us in the hearing field worry that audiologists are isolating themselves out of the market. We also worry that one of the fastest-growing segments of hearing help are PSAPs, but—as discussed in Chapter 5—audiologists don't sell them. Why are they unwilling to lend their expertise to a technology that could help millions of people begin to hear better and more easily?

Given the demographics—eight thousand baby boomers turning sixty-five every single day between 2011 and 2029, according to AARP—I'd say audiology is a growth profession. That's a lot of people who will need hearing aids and other listening technology. Whether audiologists are in private practice, at a hospital or medical center, at Costco, or employed by an Internet company, we're always going to need them.

We Need to Change the Conversation

We need to rephrase the way we talk about hearing loss. We need to talk about good hearing, hearing enhancement, and facilitating communication. We need to leave off discussing hearing in terms of levels of loss. As Wayne Staab points out, most people don't care about the degree of loss, they care about how well they communicate. The goal is to facilitate communication. Hearing aids are just one way to do that. "This goal can be accomplished with a variety of products not called hearing aids," Staab writes.[161]

In the popular mind, hearing loss is synonymous with aging. Aging is distasteful, something we'd rather not think about. Aging is also frightening: It represents the loss of youth, vitality, independence—and the inevitability of death.

We no longer venerate the elderly. The notion of a wise elder exists only in fairy tales and fantasy. In real life, our elders are too often seen as a burden. They need to be cared for—like children, but not as cute. Their teeth go bad, their hair thins, their skin mottles. And they lose their hearing.

No wonder we don't want to get there before we need to!

But the fact is that hearing loss is not just something for the elderly. We don't see those younger people with hearing loss, though, because they hide it. People with hearing loss don't want employers to know, for fear of losing their jobs. They don't want friends to know, for fear of seeming old. They may not want to acknowledge it even to themselves.

Because we aren't aware that these people are all around us, we forget that hearing loss even exists in this age group. The only people we see with hearing loss are the elderly, and even among the elderly most deny that they have any trouble with their hearing.

As a result, ignorance about hearing loss is mindboggling. Most people never even think about it, and yet it affects millions more than vision loss does. Glasses are unremarkable—and sometimes chic. Think of Sophia Loren. Could Sophia Loren make hearing aids fashionable?

If we talk about hearing loss, about how many people it affects, and how severely it can limit lives and compromise healthy aging, institutions will change. They're already beginning to.

Think about movie theaters. We wouldn't consider denying someone in a wheelchair access to a movie theater. But until very recently, people with hearing loss couldn't enjoy a movie. Now, as a result of advocacy and lawsuits, captioning devices for the hard of hearing are the law.

When I first started writing about hearing loss, just five years ago, I noticed that everywhere I went information was being broadcast through public-address systems. Flight attendants stood at boarding gates talking into a faulty mic or just shouting through a megaphone. Public transportation systems relied on conductors hollering information through public-address systems.

Now when I go to the airport or train station, information about arrivals, departures, stops, and delays is often all there in writing. Tidy, useful LED displays. Even people who can hear like them.

The New York City subway system, famous for its garbled announcements, now has information scrolling across screens in the stations and on the trains. Some stations even have fancy interactive touch screens for getting information. Remember that all the New York City subway booths are now looped. It turns out we don't really need that—the information is there in writing.

How about that information booth in the middle of Grand Central Terminal? Not quite the crossroads of the world (that's a few blocks away at Times Square) but a very busy, noisy place. What a great place for a hearing loop!

We still have a long way to go. It's amazing to me that 911

emergency systems still work only with voice calls, not text. The technology exists to text 911—all of the major cell phone providers offer it. But 92 percent of first responders around the country can't receive a 911 text. Too bad for someone like me if I happen to witness an accident or a crime and need to alert an emergency responder. I can talk, of course, but I can't answer questions, and I worry the busy operator would hang up on me.

Hearing loss itself is not an obstacle to communication. The failure in communication—in hearing—is a result instead of our personal and societal willful ignorance about hearing loss, our reluctance to acknowledge it and to treat it. The hearing aid profession's obfuscation about pricing has to change, and the costs have to come down. The hearing health professionals' internal squabbling about who has a right to sell hearing aids doesn't serve anyone. Failure to acknowledge cheaper and simpler aids to hearing, and the need for them, disserves the needy public.

But most of all, those of us with hearing loss need to speak up! Acknowledging your hearing loss, to yourself and others, is a big step toward personal acceptance. The reward is immense. But acknowledging your hearing loss is also a big step toward societal acceptance.

This book and the many resources it refers to offer much of what you need to know about hearing health, hearing loss, and hearing treatment. Hearing loss doesn't have to be the center of your life. You don't have to wonder every time you go out whether you'll be able to hear or not. Get started: Get tested, try out a PSAP if you're not ready for a hearing aid, get a hearing aid if you are ready, and add on more devices as you need them. Speak up for equality for those with imperfect hearing, advocate for looping and captions, and support those who advocate for us, like HLAA. Healthy hearing means healthier aging. Healthier aging is happier living.

GLOSSARY

There's a lot of lingo in the hearing loss world, and a lot of abbreviations. Here is a list of the most common, with definitions.

Acoustic neuroma. A benign tumor of the auditory nerve. The Mayo Clinic offers a good explanation: mayoclinic.org/diseases-conditions/acoustic-neuroma/basics/definition/con-20023851.

American Sign Language (ASL). Language used by the Culturally Deaf that involves hand signals, facial expression, and body language. It is used in the United States and Canada. Other countries have different sign languages.

Americans with Disabilities Act (ADA). Passed in 1990, it prohibits discrimination against people with disabilities. For a full explanation, see the Equal Employment Opportunity Commission's "Facts About the Americans with Disabilities Act": eeoc.gov/eeoc/publications/fs-ada.cfm.

Assistive Listening Devices (ALDs). Devices to amplify and clarify sound, especially in noise. Can be used independently or with a hearing aid or cochlear implant. See NIDCD Devices: Assistive Devices for People with Hearing, Voice, Speech, or Language Disorders: nidcd.nih.gov/health/hearing/pages/assistive-devices.aspx.

Audiogram. A graph showing the results of hearing-sensitivity tests used to determine hearing loss severity and type.

Auditory Brain Stem Implant (ABI). Similar to a cochlear implant but used when damage to the auditory nerve (see acoustic neuroma) precludes sound signals getting from the cochlea to the brain. The implant connects directly to the first auditory relay station in the brain stem. For a fuller explanation, see ASHA, Auditory Brainstem Implants, by Robert V. Shannon: asha.org/Publications/leader/2011/110315/Auditory-Brainstem-Implants.htm.

Auditory nerve. The nerve that connects the inner ear to the brain (one for each ear).

Auditory Rehabilitation. A formal or informal program for training the ear and brain after getting a hearing aid or cochlear implant. See pages 212–213.

BiCROS, CROS hearing aids. This technology is used for people with unilateral or uneven hearing loss. The BiCROS is a hearing aid–like device worn on the user's bad ear, which transmits sound wirelessly to a hearing aid on the better ear. A CROS is used if the user has normal hearing in the good ear. In that case, a wireless receiver is used to receive the transmission from the bad ear, and the user hears normally out of the good ear. A bone-anchored hearing aid can also be used in this situation.

Big Six, the. The six major hearing aid manufacturers. See Chapter 4, for a full discussion.

Bone-Anchored Hearing Aid (BAHA). Similar to a cochlear implant, the BAHA is used when damage to the outer or middle ear prevents sound signals from reaching the cochlea. The BAHA conducts sound through bone.

CART (Communication Access Real-Time Translation). Live captioning produced by a captioner or CART operator, for the use of deaf or hard of hearing people. The CART operator uses a device similar to a court reporter's stenography machine. The text, which is nearly simultaneous, is usually displayed on a screen. Remote CART uses the same principles when communication is by teleconference. The user dials in to a specific number to get the captions on a computer screen.

Centers for Medicare and Medicaid Services (CMS). Federal agency that oversees Medicare, Medicaid, and the Children's Health Insurance Program, as well as the Health Insurance Marketplace, created by the Affordable Care Act.

Cholesteatoma. An abnormal growth in the middle ear present at birth or resulting from repeated infections or trauma to the ear. A cause of conductive hearing loss.

Cochlea. The spiral cavity in the inner ear containing special sensory receptors called cochlear hair cells, which connect to the auditory nerve to transmit sound information along the auditory pathway to the brain. Damage to the hair cells is called sensorineural hearing loss and is the most common form of hearing loss. The two major causes of sensorineural loss are aging and noise exposure.

Cochlear implant (CI). An implanted device that converts sound waves to electronic signals and transmits directly to neurons on the auditory nerve. The CI bypasses the damaged outer ears and hair cells in the cochlea. For a good explanation and illustration, see the NIDCD website's page on cochlear implants: nidcd.nih.gov/health/hearing/pages/coch.aspx.

Conductive hearing loss. Hearing loss that occurs because of a blockage, injury, or malformation of the outer or middle ear, which prevents sound waves from reaching the cochlea.

Decibel (dB). See pages 24–27 for how the term is used in a hearing test. See pages 58–59 for how it is used to measure environmental noise.

Direct to consumer sales. Also called Direct to Consumer Marketing. Term used for the sale of hearing aids or other devices directly to the consumer rather than through an audiologist or hearing aid dispenser.

Dizziness. A feeling of lightheadedness and imbalance, where your surroundings do NOT feel as though they are moving. Compare to *vertigo*.

Ear mold. A silicone-based mold of the outer ear, used to determine the proper fit for an in-the-ear hearing aid.

ENT. Ear, nose, and throat doctor. Usually an otolaryngologist.

FM system. A personal FM system consists of a transmitter/microphone, which a speaker uses, and a receiver, used by the person with hearing loss. *FM* stands for frequency modulation, and the sound is transmitted by radio waves. If you wear hearing aids or a cochlear implant, you can turn on the telecoil setting to augment the sound. If you don't have a hearing aid, you can use a headset.

Frequency. The physical frequency at which air vibrates, which we experience as pitch, measured in hertz, at which a tone is heard. A birdcall or a standard telephone ring are high frequency tones. Water dripping or a large dog's bark are low frequency tones. Speech sounds vary across the frequency spectrum. An audiogram will show how well you hear at each frequency between 125 and 8,000 Hz. Humans can hear up to 20,000 Hz.

Hertz (Hz). A unit for measuring frequency. *Webster's New Collegiate Dictionary* describes a hertz (named after German physicist Heinrich

Hertz) as "equal to one cycle per second." High frequency sounds are measured as 4,000–5,000 cycles per second; low frequency as 125 to 500 cycles per second.

Hyperacusis. An unusual sensitivity to sounds, which may make it difficult to tolerate everyday sounds.

Induction Loop System. An assistive listening system in which a room or area is wired to pick up and transmit sound to a listener. See Chapter 20 for a full discussion of hearing loops.

Infrared device. An assistive listening system used in many theaters to transmit sound to the listener by means of infrared light waves. The listener wears either earphones or a neckloop receiver and a headset. If you have a T-coil in your hearing aid, the neckloop receiver will send the sound to your hearing aid via the T-coil setting, making the headset unnecessary. Infrared systems are also used for watching TV. (Your TV remote works using infrared technology.)

Lip-reading. This is the now outdated term for speech-reading.

Looping. See Induction Loop System.

Ménière's disease. A disease of the vestibular system in the inner ear that can cause hearing loss, balance problems, fullness in the ear, and tinnitus. It is idiopathic, meaning the cause is not known.

Neckloop. A general term used to describe anything worn around the neck. Most often it refers to the receiver used with an FM system or an infrared system. Bluetooth streamers are also sometimes neckloops.

Noise-induced hearing loss. Noise-induced hearing loss, similar to age-related hearing loss, is often a symmetrical loss in both ears. It can be asymmetrical if the cause was a gunshot near one ear or another loud sound from one side. It is often progressive, and noise-related hearing loss can accelerate age-related loss. Together the two are responsible for most hearing loss.

Occupational Safety and Health Administration (OSHA). A federal agency that regulates workplace safety, including noise levels.

Otolaryngology. A medical specialty concerned with the ear, nose, and throat. An otolaryngologist may also be an **otologist**, with a specialty in inner ear pathology, or a **neurotologist**, a specialist in the parts of the nervous system having to do with the ear. The overall title of the medical department is often the **Department of Otolaryngology—Head and Neck Surgery**.

Otosclerosis. A disease of the bones of the middle ear, affecting the stapes. The principal symptom is gradual hearing loss. This is conductive loss, because the sound waves are blocked from reaching the cochlea. "What You Should Know About Otosclerosis," by the American Academy of Otolaryngology—Head and Neck Surgery, is a very clear discussion: entnet.org/?q=node/1316.

Otoscope. An instrument, with a light and magnifying lenses, used to examine the eardrum and the external ear canal.

Ototoxin. Anything that can damage hearing. See pages 64–65 for a full discussion.

Personal Sound Amplification Product. See PSAP.

Presbycusis. Age-related hearing loss.

PSAP (Personal Sound Amplification Product). A hearing aid–like device that has not been approved by the FDA for use to correct hearing loss. See full discussion in Chapter 5.

Pure-tone threshold. This is the lowest level at which you can detect a sound at a single frequency at least 50 percent of the time. The pure-tone test, which measures this, is the basic hearing test.

Receiver. In hearing loss, anything used to receive signals transmitted by FM, infrared, or Bluetooth. Usually worn as a neckloop.

Rehabilitation Engineering Research Center (RERC). See Resources.

Reverberation. An acoustics term referring to the reflected sound from the surfaces in a space such as an auditorium. Some degree of reverberation is desirable, in that it helps distribution of sound around the space. For people with hearing loss, a space with a lot of reverberation can make it difficult to understand speech or sounds.

Sensorineural hearing loss. Hearing loss caused by damage to the cochlea or the auditory nerve. Most commonly, the damage is to the hair cells. Sensorineural hearing loss can usually be treated with hearing aids or cochlear implants.

Signal-to-noise ratio (SNR). A measure of how loud a desired sound needs to be to be heard over background noise.

Speech banana. The pattern on an audiogram showing where most speech sounds occur. If your hearing falls below the decibel level needed to hear at a certain frequency (for instance, if you need the sound turned higher than 40 decibels to hear sounds in the high frequencies), you will have trouble distinguishing letters like *th* and *s*. For a diagram of the speech banana, go to listeningandspoken language.org/SpeechBanana/. Or simply Google "speech banana" and you'll see a variety of illustrations.

Speech-in-noise test. This measures your signal-to-noise ratio and tells an audiologist how to program the different frequencies of a hearing aid or cochlear implant.

Speech-reading, also called lip-reading. Speech-reading involves watching not only the speaker's lips but also facial expressions and body language. It is most effective when used in conjunction with some degree of hearing.

Streamer. Device that picks up signals from an audio source and transmits them wirelessly to hearing aids or a cochlear implant. Typically used with TV, computer, stereo system, or cell phone. The streamer is usually worn as a neckloop.

Sudden hearing loss. Also known as Sudden Deafness, Sudden Hearing Loss (SHL) or Sudden Sensorineural Hearing loss (SSHL).

The loss of 30 decibels of hearing in three contiguous frequencies over seventy-two hours or less. For more information, see pages 66–68. The cause is often unknown, in which case it is called Idiopathic Sudden Sensorineural Hearing Loss, or ISSHL.

T-coil. See Telecoil.

Teleaudiology. A branch of telemedicine that provides audiology services to people in remote areas.

Telecoil. A small copper wire in a hearing aid or cochlear implant that is activated by flipping a dial to access the program. For a full description and uses of a telecoil, see Chapter 18.

Transmitter. Used with FM systems and other wireless devices, the transmitter sends signals to the receiver, usually worn as a neckloop.

Tympanogram. The result of a test to measure the health and flexibility of the eardrum (the tympanic membrane).

Vertigo. In medical terminology, a form of dizziness in which you have the sensation that you or your environment is spinning or moving. True vertigo is caused by an imbalance in the vestibular system, and is often accompanied by nystagmus (an involuntary eye movement, which feels like the eyes are snapping back and forth) and nausea. It is sometimes a symptom of Ménière's disease or other vestibular disorders and can be difficult to control.

BPPV (benign paroxysmal positional vertigo) is a common form of vertigo that results from sudden head movements. It can usually be controlled by exercises taught by a doctor or physical therapist. See the American Institute of Balance for more information: dizzy.com/dizzines_and_equilibrium.htm.

Vestibular system. Sensory system adjacent to the cochlea that includes two sets of semicircular canals. These contain special receptors for motion, equilibrium, and spatial orientation. Signals from the system travel along a special branch of the auditory nerve to the brain. The balance and auditory systems are closely related.

RESOURCES

Organizations and Websites

American Academy of Audiology (AAA)

American Doctors of Audiology (ADA)

American Speech-Language-Hearing Association (ASHA)

Association of Late-Deafened Adults (ALDA)

Better Hearing Institute (BHI)

Canadian Hard of Hearing Association (CHHA)

Center for Hearing Loss Help

Consumer Electronics Association (CEA); represents PSAP
    manufacturers

Hearing Aid Forums: hearingaidforums.com/

Hearing Industries Association (HIA); represents hearing aid
    manufacturers

Hearing Loss Association of America (HLAA)

IDA Institute

International Hearing Society

National Association of the Deaf (NAD)

RERC: hearingresearch.org/index.php

Ross Hearing Center: rosshearingcenter.com

Sound Strategy, Cynthia Compton-Conley: soundstrategy.com/tutorials

Books

These books address adult-onset hearing loss. There are many books
on Deafness (by Harlan Lane, among others), books dealing with the
causes and kinds of hearing problems in children, books about tinnitus
treatments, etc. I have not included these. This is a highly selective list,
including only books I have read and admired.

Textbooks

Kaplan, Harriet, Scott J. Bally, and Carol Garretson. *Speechreading: A
    Way to Improve Understanding.* 2d ed., rev. ed. Washington, D.C.:
    Gallaudet University Press, 1995.

Lustig, Tracy A., Steve Olson, Forum on Aging, Disability and Independence, National Research Council, and Institute of Medicine. *Hearing Loss and Healthy Aging: Workshop Summary.* Washington, D.C.: National Academies Press, 2014.

Montano, Joseph J., and Jaclyn B. Spitzer. *Adult Audiologic Rehabilitation.* 2d ed. San Diego: Plural Publishing, 2014.

Niparko, John D., ed. *Cochlear Implants: Principles & Practices.* 2d ed. Philadelphia: Lippincott Williams & Wilkins, April 2009.

Books for the General Reader

Alexander, Rebecca, with Sascha Alper. *Not Fade Away.* New York: Gotham Books, 2014.

Bell, Cece. *El Deafo.* New York: Amulet Books, 2014. (Technically for kids but good for anyone.)

Chorost, Michael. *Rebuilt: My Journey Back to the Hearing World.* Boston: Houghton Mifflin, 2006.

Groves, Shana. *Confessions of a Lip Reading Mom.* Colby, KS: CrossRiver Media Group, 2013.

Hannan, Gael. *The Way I Hear It: A Life with Hearing Loss.* 2015.

Harvey, Michael A. *Odyssey of Hearing Loss: Tales of Triumph.* San Diego: DawnSign Press, 2004.

Horowitz, Seth S. *The Universal Sense: How Hearing Shapes the Mind.* New York: Bloomsbury, 2012.

Lodge, David. *Deaf Sentence.* New York: Viking, 2008 (Fiction).

Myers, David G. *A Quiet World: Living with Hearing Loss.* New Haven, CT: Yale University Press, 2000.

Romoff, Arlene. *Hear Again: Back to Life with a Cochlear Implant.* New York: League for the Hard of Hearing, 2000.

———. *Listening Closely: A Journey to Bilateral Hearing.* Watertown, MA: Imagine! Publishing, 2011.

Shea, Gerald. *Song Without Words: Discovering My Deafness Halfway Through Life.* Boston: Da Capo Press, 2013.

Swiller, Josh. *The Unheard: A Memoir of Deafness and Africa.* New York: Henry Holt, 2007.

Blogs

"The Better Hearing Consumer." Gael Hannan. Hearing Health & Technology Matters. hearinghealthmatters.org/betterhearingconsumer/about-gael-hannan/.

"Healthy Hearing." Katherine Bouton. AARP online. blog.aarp.org/author/aarpkbouton/.

"Hear Better with Hearing Loss." Katherine Bouton. hearbetterwithhearingloss.wordpress.com.

"Hear the Music." Marshall Chasin. Hearing Health & Technology Matters. hearinghealthmatters.org/hearthemusic/.

"Hearing Economics." Holly Hosford-Dunn. Hearing Health & Technology Matters. hearinghealthmatters.org/hearingeconomics/.

"Hearing News Watch." David Kirkwood. Hearing Health & Technology Matters. hearinghealthmatters.org/hearingnewswatch/.

"Lipreading Mom." Shanna Groves. lipreadingmom.com/.

"Wayne's World." Wayne Staab. Hearing Health & Technology Matters. hearinghealthmatters.org/waynesworld/.

"What I Hear." Katherine Bouton. *Psychology Today* website. psychologytoday.com/blog/what-i-hear.

Online Newsletters and Magazines

Some are also published on paper.

The Hearing Journal. journals.lww.com/thehearingjournal/pages/default.aspx.

Hearing Loss Magazine. For members of the Hearing Loss Association of America. hearingloss.org/content/hearing-loss-magazine.

The Hearing Review. hearingreview.com/.

The Journal at Hearing Health & Technology Matters. hearinghealthmatters.org/.

RERC: Rehabilitation Engineering Research Centers. resnaprojects.org/nattap/at/rercs.html.

NOTES

Part One: Facing Facts

Chapter 1, I Don't Have Hearing Loss. I Just Can't Hear You.

1 *Encyclopedia of Mental Disorders*, minddisorders.com/Del-Fi/Denial.html.

2 Sergei Kochkin, "The Impact of Treated Hearing Loss on Quality of Life," Better Hearing Institute.

3 These numbers vary from source to source. According to betterhearing.org, for instance, "The majority (65%) of people with hearing loss are younger than age 65." betterhearing.org/hearingpedia/prevalence-hearing-loss.

4 hearingreview.com/2013/07/hr-blog-has-costco-become-king-of-us-hearing-aid-retailing-2/.

5 Hi HealthInnovations Program, UnitedHealthcare, hihealthinnovations.com/medicare.

6 AARP Hearing Aid discounts, aarphealthcare.com/insurance/hearing-care-program.html?intcmp=MBCHHEATAB1POS4.

7 blog.aarp.org/2015/01/21/talking-about-hearing-loss-to-someone-who-doesnt-want-to-listen/.

Chapter 2, Get It Tested

8 You can also get a hearing screening at community centers and health fairs—especially those targeted at seniors—at a speech-language pathologist, or from a hearing instrument specialist who sells hearing aids.

9 These might include uneven hearing loss, hearing loss in just one ear, or hearing loss that didn't follow patterns that might suggest age- or noise-related hearing loss.

Chapter 3, Your First Audiologist Appointment

10 asha.org/findpro/.

11 Owned retail channels are as follows: Phonak: Hearing Planet, Connect Hearing; GN ReSound: Beltone, McDonald, Hearing Minnesota; Oticon: AHAA, Avada, Hearing Life, Accuquest; Siemens: HearUSA; Widex: Revive, AMEar; Starkey: All American Hearing.

12 http://www.asha.org/aud/Know-the-Facts/.

13 "HR 2013 Hearing Aid Dispenser Survey: Dispensing in the Age of Internet and Big Box Retailers," *Hearing Review*, April 8, 2014.

14 Here is a list of the functions audiologists perform, followed by a list of what hearing aid specialists are qualified for:
Audiologists:
Comprehensive evaluations including hearing, speech understanding, middle ear function, inner ear and auditory nerve function. Diagnostic tests for balance/dizziness disorders. Auditory-processing evaluations for infants, children, and adults. Fitting and verification of hearing instruments and assistive listening devices. Design, selection, installation and monitoring of classroom amplification systems.

Rehabilitation therapies. Earwax management. Tinnitus evaluation/management. Counseling. Development of hearing conservation programs. Research.

Hearing aid specialists:

Basic hearing tests exclusively for the purpose of selling hearing aids to adults. Hearing aid fitting and sales. Assistive devices.

15 Wallhagen is also the current chair of the Board of Trustees of the Hearing Loss Association of America. The 2014 conference, sponsored by the Institute of Medicine and the National Research Council, brought together many experts from the fields of hearing loss and gerontology, and I will cite this meeting several times in the course of the book. A summary of the two-day workshop is available from the National Academies Press.

16 Much of the information on testing comes from ASHA's guidelines for audiologists. They are far more detailed and can be found at asha.org/policy/GL2005-00014/.

17 An audiologist who read this passage commented that everyone with hearing loss answers this one like that.

18 For information about Dr. Bauman and The Center for Hearing Loss Help, go to hearinglosshelp.com/aboutus/meetdirector.htm.

19 For more about decibel levels and percentages, read Neil Bauman's very clear explanation on Hearing Loss Help: hearinglosshelp.com/articles/decibelsvspercent .htm.

Chapter 4, Hearing Aids: So Many Choices

20 David Kirkwood is the former editor of the *Hearing Journal*. His blog on *Hearing Health & Technology Matters* is the source of much invaluable information. hearinghealthmatters.org/hearingviews/david-kirkwood-bio/.

21 Terminology differs from one source of information to another. For this section, I've relied on *Consumer Reports*'s "Hearing Aid Buying Guide," AARP's "Consumer Guide to Hearing Aids," Hearing Planet's "Hearing Aid Buyer's Guide," and the FDA's "Types of Hearing Aids." Where the sources agree, I've simply stated the information. Where they disagree or one offers information that the others lack, I've noted the source.

22 The 2014 *Consumer Reports* prices tend to be slightly lower, because they are based on a 2008 survey. *CR* gives a price range from $185 to $2,700 per aid.

23 hearingreview.com/2015/01/hearing-aid-sales-increase-4-8-2014-rics-continue-market-domination.

24 AARP's "Consumer Guide to Hearing Aids," assets.aarp.org/www.aarp.org_/articles/ health/docs/hearing_guide.pdf.

25 Dr. Mark Ross, "Invisible Extended Wear Hearing Aids," hearingresearch.org/ross/ hearing_aids/invisible_extended_wear_hearing_aids.php.

26 Here are a couple of places to read about the Esteem: leahlefler.hubpages.com/hub/ The-Esteem-Hearing-Implant-An-Invisible-Hearing-Aid-Alternative, and Audiology Online: audiologyonline.com/articles/the-esteem-middle-ear-implant-12780. Note that the author is an audiologist with Envoy Medical.

27 "Unbundling Hearing Aid Sales," ASHA News, .asha.org/PRPSpecificTopic.aspx?folder id=8589934966&section=Key_Issues.

28 *The Hearing Review*, hearingreview.com/, a magazine and online publication for hearing-health-care professionals and hearing aid providers. The editor is Karl Strom.

29 David Kirkwood discussed the consolidation in a 2011 column: hearinghealthmatters .org/hearingviews/2011/though-the-big-six-hearing-aid-makers-are-still-intact-consolidation-isnt-over-in-the-hearing-industry/.

30 See a list of states and their specific policies at hearingloss.org/content/state-hearing-health-insurance-mandates.

31 militaryaudiology.org/site/.

32 For state vocational rehabilitation agencies: hearingloss.org/content/state-agencies.

33 You can read more about these plans in the *Hearing Review*'s "10 Tips for Hearing Aid Financing," October 31, 2014.

Chapter 5, The Not-Ready-for-a-Hearing-Aid "Hearing Aid"

34 "FDA Draft Guidance Report on Regulatory Requirements for Hearing Aid Devices and Personal Sound Amplification Products," November 7, 2013, fda.gov/ medicaldevices/deviceregulationandguidance/guidancedocuments/ucm373461.htm.

35 David Kirkwood, "FDA's Proposed New PSAP Policy Draws Mixed Response, but Mostly Opposed," Hearing News Watch at *Hearing Health & Technology Matters*, February 14, 2014.

36 Statement from the Hearing Loss Association of America on PSAPs, October 14, 2014.

37 Gina Shaw, "PSAPs: To Beat Them or to Join Them?" March 2014, journals.lww.com/ thehearingjournal/Fulltext/2014/03000/PSAPs___To_Beat_Them,_or_to_Join_ Them_.1.aspx.

38 hearinghealthmatters.org/.

39 Most hearing aids also have a thirty-day return policy. Consumer groups like the Hearing Loss Association of America recommend a sixty-day return policy.

40 See Wayne Staab, "HA Distribution VII—PSAP, ALD, or Hearing Aid," *Hearing Health & Technology Matters*, hearinghealthmatters.org/waynesworld/2013/ha-distribution-vii-psap-ald-or-hearing-aid/.

41 "Soundhawk Smart Listening System: A Hearing Helper," nytimes.com/2014/11/20/ technology/personaltech/soundhawk-smart-listening-system-a-hearing-helper.html.

42 Judith Graham, "When Hearing Aids Won't Do," newoldage.blogs.nytimes .com/2013/06/12/when-hearing-aids-wont-do/.

Chapter 6, How Did This Happen?

43 Hearing Loss and Healthy Aging, see Note 15.

44 Pamela Mason of ASHA, quoted by the BBC, "How to Cut Noise in a Plane Cabin," February 26, 2014, bbc.com/future/story/20140226-tricks-for-a-peaceful-flight.

45 "Which NFL Team Has Fans Loud Enough to Trigger Earthquakes?" blog.aarp .org/2015/01/15/which-nfl-team-has-fans-loud-enough-to-trigger-earthquakes/.

46 The Sight & Hearing Association at the University of Minnesota does an annual survey of toys. audiologyonline.com/releases/sight-hearing-association-releases-annual-12388-12388.

47 In the decade ending in 2010, there were 840,865 service-related cases of tinnitus, and 701,760 cases of hearing loss. Post-traumatic stress disorder was third, at 501,280. I wrote about hearing problems in the military at greater length in *Shouting Won't Help*: 232–236.

48 "Hearing Aids and Cognitive Decline," M. K. Pichora-Fuller et al., in *Hearing Aids: The Brain Connection*, guest editor Kelley L. Tremblay, PhD, 2013: 311.

49 nidcd.nih.gov/health/statistics/pages/quick.aspx.

50 This information is from the American Academy of Otolaryngology—Head and Neck Surgery website on genes and hearing loss: entnet.org/content/genes-and-hearing-loss.

51 Sujana S. Chandrasekhar, MD, "Otosclerosis," newyorkotology.com/patient-information/symptoms/otosclerosis/.

52 Two excellent sources on Sudden Hearing Loss:

> NIDCD, nidcd.nih.gov/health/hearing/pages/sudden.aspx.

> Massachusetts Eye and Ear Infirmary, Steven D. Rauch, masseyeandear.org/for-patients/patient-guide/patient-education/diseases-and-conditions/sudden-deafness/, updated 2011.

53 Marshall Chasin, AuD, "Obituary: The CROS Hearing Aid (1964–2014)," *Hearing Review,* May 2014.

Chapter 7, Practice, Practice, Practice

54 "Does Your Loved One Need a Hearing Test?" October 8, 2014, aarp.org/health/conditions-treatments/info-2014/help-a-loved-one-with-hearing-loss.html?intcmp=AE-MIV-HEARINGRC-LIVING-WELL.

55 healthyhearing.com/content/faqs/Hearing-aids/Fitting/31057-Phonemic-regression. One 2015 study found that cognition actually improved in older adults with profound hearing loss who received cochlear implants followed by intensive auditory rehabilitation. Cochlear Implants found to reverse cognitive decline in elderly patients. blog.aarp.org/2015/03/26/cochlear-implants-shown-to-reverse-cognitive-decline.

56 I wrote about this case for *The New York Times* Op-Ed page. nytimes.com/2015/03/28/opinion/cops-with-hearing-aids.html. I also wrote a longer piece in *Hearing Loss Magazine*, May/June 2015 issue.

57 John Greer Clark and Carissa Maatman Weiser, "Patient Motivation in Adult Audiologic Rehabilitation," Chapter 11 in *Adult Audiologic Rehabilitation*, 2d ed., by Joseph J. Montano and Jaclyn B. Spitzer. (Plural Publishing), 207.

58 chchearing.org/.

59 angelsound.tigerspeech.com/.

60 LACE, neurotone.com/lace-interactive-listening-program.

Part Two: Love and Work

Chapter 8, Family Matters

61 Melissa Echalier, "In It Together: The Impact of Hearing Loss on Personal Relationships," RNID, IDA Institute, idainstitute.com/fileadmin/user_upload/

documents/In%20It%20Together%20-%20Impact%20on%20Personal%20
Relationships.pdf.

62 "The Better Hearing Consumer," *Hearing Health & Technology Matters*,
hearinghealthmatters.org/betterhearingconsumer/about-gael-hannan/.

63 deaf-insight.com/ask-lipreading-mom/help-i-suspect-my-spouse-has-hearing-loss.

64 Rebecca Alexander, *Not Fade Away* (Gotham Books, 2014): 288–289.

65 livestrong.com/article/241930-the-best-baby-monitors-for-the-hearing-impaired/.

66 michdhh.org/assistive_devices/baby_cry_monitor.html.

67 Existing systems for hearing things like the doorbell—Silent Call, Sonic Alert, or
Alertmaster—can be wired to the baby monitor. You can also tune the monitor for
sensitivity. If you want to know when your baby coos and murmurs, you can turn
up the sensitivity. If you live in an apartment building, you'll also want a higher
frequency model, to prevent interference from other apartments, and also from
other wireless devices in your own home. The Michigan website (see Note 66) also
lists places to buy baby monitors. Harris Communications offers many devices for
the deaf and hard of hearing, including baby monitors. (It also sells fire alarms for
the hard of hearing, essential for anyone with a high frequency loss, which is where
conventional alarms sound. For people with severe hearing loss, these should include
a bed shaker in addition to a strobe light.)

68 Here's one study: aut.researchgateway.ac.nz/bitstream/handle/10292/900/WardA.
pdf?sequence=3.

Chapter 9, Dating: Who, How, and When to Tell

69 Sergei Kochkin.

70 Cochlear Implant Online was founded in 2001 by Rachel Chaikof, a cochlear
implant user who was fourteen at the time. Her sister Jessica is a guest blogger:
cochlearimplantonline.com/site/dating-relationships-marriage-and-hearing-loss-full-
survey-results/.

71 *International Journal of Impotence Research/The Journal of Sexual Medicine*. February 15,
2007, nature.com/ijir/journal/v19/n4/full/3901547a.html%3Fref%3Ddod-jptc
.org?message=remove&ref=dod-jptc.org.

Chapter 10, You Gotta Have Friends

72 Katherine Bouton, "Eighty Years Along, a Longevity Study Still Has Ground to Cover,"
nytimes.com/2011/04/19/science/19longevity.html?pagewanted=print.

73 The New York City chapter has a continually updated list of venues on its website,
helpful not only to residents but also to visitors with hearing loss: hearinglossnyc.org/
wp-content/uploads/2014/09/Web-Looped-NYC-venues.pdf.

74 HLAA State Organizations and Chapters: hearingloss.org/content/hlaa-chapters-and-
state-organizations.

75 ALDA Chapter and Group Directory: alda.org/resources/chapter-and-group.

Chapter 11, The Job Search

76 "How to Write a Resume: Dos and Don'ts," cbsnews.com/news/how-to-write-a-
resume-dos-and-donts/.

77 "Job Searches, Discrimination and Questions About How and When to Disclose," hearinglossboston.org/job-searches-discrimination-and-questions-about-how-and-when-to-disclose/.

78 "My Disability: To Disclose or Not to Disclose," teaching.monster.com/careers/articles/4332-my-disability-to-disclose-or-not-to-disclose.

79 There's a link to the PDF on the HLAA website: hearingloss.org/content/employment.

80 You can read the settlement at: dralegal.org/sites/dralegal.org/files/casefiles/154ordersettlement.pdf.

Chapter 12, Once You Get the Job

81 What's 2.4 GHz? Here's a good explanation from Wired: wired.com/2010/09/wireless-explainer/.

82 See "Quandary of Hidden Disabilities: Conceal or Reveal?" which I wrote for *The New York Times* in 2013.

83 research.gallandet.edu/demographics/deaf-employed-zoll.pdf.

84 Donna A. Morere, "Reading and the Deaf or Hard of Hearing Child," *Reading in 2010: A Comprehensive Review of a Changing Field* (Nova Science Publishers, 2010).

85 The book includes a very interesting discussion on deaf and hard of hearing and education. Chapters 18–20 focus on learning and reading.

Chapter 13, Mid-Career Hearing Loss, or, My Mistakes

86 See Chapter 23 for a more detailed discussion of hearing loss and cognitive stress.

87 You can find out more about TDF's Theatre Accessibility Program at tdf.org/nyc/33/TDFAccessibilityPrograms.

88 Every harried working woman should read her hilarious and insightful *Bossypants*.

Part Three: Travel and Leisure

Chapter 14, Flying and Lodging

89 nad.org/issues/transportation-and-travel/hotels-and-motels.

90 ada.gov/hotelcombr.htm.

Chapter 15, On the Road

91 hearinglosshelp.com/articles/drivesafely.htm.

92 lipreadingmom.com/2014/08/12/when-you-get-pulled-over-and-cant-hear-the-pearl-pearson-story/.

93 google.com/search?q=deaf+driver+visor+card&tbm=isch&tbo=u&source=univ&sa=X&ei=PvLoU4axOMmKyASHi4CwAg&ved=0CCAQsAQ&biw=1024&bih=648.

94 aclu.org/know-your-deaf-rights-what-do-when-dealing-police.

95 hearinglosshelp.com/articles/visorcards.htm.

Chapter 16, Dining Out

96 elevatingsound.com/acoustics-is-bound-to-become-the-next-big-thing-in-providing-a-great-dining-experience/.

97 Adam Platt, "Why Restaurants Are Louder than Ever," July 22, 2013, newyork .grubstreet.com/2013/07/adam-platt-on-loud-restaurants.html.

98 You can watch a video discussion of the Comal installation at youtube.com/watch?v=f-QFK-IpkM8.

99 "Hi-tech System Lets Restaurant Set Noise Level," sfgate.com/business/article/High-tech-system-lets-restaurant-set-noise-level-3554029.php.

100 Interesting interview with a number of chefs about noise in restaurants: eater .com/2012/8/24/6551933/chefs-weigh-in-on-loud-and-noisy-restaurants.

Part Four: When Hearing Aids Aren't Enough

Chapter 18, Roger and Me: Assistive Technology

101 "Market Perception of the Impact of Inductively Looped Venues on the Utility of Their Hearing Devices." *The Hearing Review.* September 24, 2014.

102 nidcd.nih.gov/health/hearing/pages/assistive-devices.aspx.

103 Sound Strategy: soundstrategy.com/tutorials.

104 Compton-Conley discusses these devices in a video of a talk she delivered in 2014: iom.edu/Activities/PublicHealth/HearingLossAging/2014-JAN-13/Day%202/ Session%20V/22-Compton-Conley-Video.aspx.

105 A 2014 *Hearing Review* study found that 71.5 percent of hearing aids have a telecoil. If you eliminate the tiny CIC models (Completely in the Canal), the percentage goes up to 80.5 percent. Surprisingly, given the assistive listening devices that are increasingly available, which often rely on a telecoil to transmit sound to the hearing aid, this percentage isn't much higher than that found in a similar, but smaller, study in 2009–10. That study found that 69 percent had telecoils. In some hearing aid models, the telecoil is found in a remote control or in a streamer, a small gateway device that also gives the user access to cell phone and TV signals.

106 The Hearing Aid Compatibility Act of 1988 (HAC Act) requires that the Federal Communications Commission ensure that *all* telephones manufactured or imported for use in the United States after August 1989, and all "essential" telephones, are hearing aid compatible. "Essential" telephones are defined as "coin-operated telephones, telephones provided for emergency use and other telephones frequently needed for use by persons using such hearing aids." "Essential" phones might include workplace phones, phones in confined settings (like hospitals and nursing homes), and phones in hotel and motel rooms. Secure phones (approved by the U.S. government to transmit classified or sensitive conversations) and phones used with public mobile and private radio services are exempt from the HAC Act. See fcc.gov/ guides/hearing-aid-compatibility-wireline-telephones.

107 betterhearing.org/hearingpedia/hearing-aid-compatible-cell-phones.

108 The Center for Hearing Loss Help has a good write-up on cell phones: hearinglosshelp .com/articles/hacphones.htm.

109 ASHA on hearing aid compatible cell phones: asha.org/public/hearing/Hearing-Aids-and-Cell-Phones/.

110 hearingloss.org/content/telephones-and-mobile-devices.

111 tdf.org/nyc/33/TDFAccessibilityPrograms.

112 Technology for the Enhancement of Face-to-Face Communication: soundstrategy
.com/content/technology-enhancement-face-face-communication#wireless-hearing-
aid.

113 A clear explanation of FM systems can be found at hearinglink.org/fm-systems.

114 williamssound.com/digiwave/.

115 fedretire.net/how-to-manage-your-own-hearing-health-care-2/.

116 audiologyonline.com/releases/new-phonak-technology-allows-people-12906.

117 audiologyonline.com/interviews/new-study-shows-phonak-226-13161.

118 Tammara Stender, AuD, "Beyond Connectivity." This article is about the ReSound
LiNX, which offers direct connectivity to the iPhone, iPad, and iPod Touch.

119 cnn.com/2014/03/04/tech/innovation/apple-resound-hearing-aids/.

120 Farhad Manjoo, "Conjuring Images of a Bionic Future," *The New York Times*, April 23,
2014.

121 Anthony Wing Kosner, "Made for iPhone Hearing Aids: Hands on with Halo, a
Mission-Critical Wearable," forbes.com/sites/anthonykosner/2014/08/16/made-for-
iphone-hearing-aids-hands-on-with-halo-a-mission-critical-wearable/.
    The *Forbes* article includes details about other Made for iPhone brands:
"Although Apple lists seven distinct compatible devices on its iOS hearing aid page
(Audibel A3i, Audigy AGXsp, Beltone First, MicroTech Kinnect, NuEar iSDS,
ReSound LiNX, and Starkey Halo), Fabry tells me that there are actually only two
distinctly different Made for iPhone products on the market: Starkey's Halo/TruLink
and GN ReSound's LiNX. Beltone's product is a rebranded version of the LiNX and
the other four are rebranded versions of Starkey's TruLink. All of the Starkey devices
use the TruLink app and ReSound and Beltone use color-branded versions of the
LiNX, and truthfully both apps are quite similar. This is probably a reflection of the
limited nature of the APIs that Apple has made available. As with all things Apple,
this limitation is supposed to assure the quality of the user experience, but I am
hoping for some more innovative functionality from Apple and its partners."

122 hearinglosshelp.com/articles/firesafety.htm.

123 soundstrategy.com/tutorials/how-alerting-technology-can-keep-you-and-your-family-
safe-and-add-convenience-your-life.

Chapter 19, Read My Lips!

124 "Learning to Speechread (Lipread)," April 19, 2014, is the most recent and recaps much
of what can be found in earlier posts. See hearinglosshelp.com/weblog/category/
coping-strategies/speechreading.

125 "4 Ears, 4 Eyes: Misadventures in Deafness." 4ears4eyes.com/2013/01/how-to-be-
lipreader-friendly.html.

126 The publisher is Gallaudet University Press. This is a 1985 paperback in a revised
second edition.

127 Gallaudet Resources to Develop Speechreading Skills: gallaudet.edu/clerc_center/
information_and_resources/info_to_go/language_and_literacy/spoken_language_
development/resources_to_develop_speechreading_skills.html.

Gallaudet's recommendations include several DVD/book combinations, including *I See What You Say.* You can also order this on Amazon.com for $58.66. The Amazon user reviews are mixed. Another Gallaudet recommendation is *Read My Lips*, six VHS videocassettes. I wasn't able to find these offered in a more updated format.

128 deafness.about.com/cs/communication/a/lipreading.htm.

Chapter 20, What the Heck Is a Hearing Loop?

129 Richard Einhorn, quoted in "A Hearing Aid That Cuts Out All the Clatter," *The New York Times*, October 23, 2011, nytimes.com/2011/10/24/science/24loops.html?_r=0.

130 R. Magann Faivre, F. Ismail, J. Sterkens, T. Thunder, and K. Chung, "The Effects of Hearing Loop Systems on Speech Understanding and Sound Quality in Real-World Listening Environments." Poster session presented at: Northern Illinois University Audiology Clinic, NIU Speech and Hearing Clinic; May 9, 2013.

131 The Metropolitan Opera (whose singers do not wear body mics) offers headsets, which pick up sound from a microphone above the orchestra. These are high-quality mics, but users report that the sound doesn't translate well through the headphones.

I prefer to listen with my hearing aid and implant and catch as much as I can. I have the hearing aid at a normal volume, because it's better at discerning pitch and music in general, and the cochlear implant, which is notoriously bad with music, turned down just low enough to give me balance. I have been to HD performances of the Met Opera—the sound there, through loudspeakers in a theater or auditorium, is good. I wonder if the Met broadcasts are done at any theaters that have looping. That would be fabulous.

Chapter 21, Cochlear Implants

132 hearinglosshelp.com/weblog/finding-a-good-cochlear-implant-surgeon.php.

133 "I Look So I Can Hear," funnyoldlife.wordpress.com/cochlear-implants/choosing-a-brand/.

134 FDA Approves First Implantable Hearing Device for Adults with a Certain Kind of Hearing loss, fda.gov/newsevents/newsroom/pressannouncements/ucm389860.htm.

135 cochlear.com/wps/wcm/connect/us/recipients/baha-3/baha-3-basics/basics.

136 oticonmedical.com/.

137 sophono.com/2011/05/sophono-receives-clearance-from-fda-to-market-implantable-alpha-1m-to-united-states/.

138 hearing.health.mil/DiagnosisTreatment/TreatmentOptions/BoneAnchoredImplant .aspx.

139 medgadget.com/2013/12/cochlear-limited-receives-fda-approval-for-magnetic-bone-conduction-hearing-device.html.

140 Here's the relevant paragraph from the proposal:

c. Proposed clarification of the statutory Medicare hearing aid coverage exclusion stipulated at section 1862(a)(7) of the Act. This proposed rule proposes to clarify the scope of the Medicare coverage exclusion for hearing aids and withdraw coverage of bone-anchored hearing aids.

"This proposal would not have a significant fiscal impact on the Medicare program, because the Medicare program expenditures for bone-anchored hearing aids during the period CY2005 through CY2013 are less than $9,000,000. This proposed rule, if finalized, would provide further guidance about coverage of DME (Durable Medical Equipment) with regard to the statutory hearing aid exclusion. The proposed rule, if finalized, would leave unchanged coverage of cochlear implants and brain stem implants, which are not considered hearing aids."

141 The home page of Pisoni's Speech Research Laboratory will lead you to many of his publications: iu.edu/~srlweb/people/david-pisoni/.

142 Here's the link to the program: neurotone.com/lace-interactive-listening-program.

143 "Cochlear Implant Rehabilitation: It's Not Just for Kids!" cochlear.com/wps/wcm/connect/ad6e0aa3-b176-4bf1-9e5e-8d99e67a0781/product_cochlearimplant_rehabilitationresources_teensandadults_cochlearimplantrehabilitation itsnotjustforkids_en_433kb.pdf?MOD=AJPERES&CONVERT_TO=url&CACHEID=ad6e0aa3-b176-4bf1-9e5e-8d99e67a0781.

144 The Listening Room: hearingjourney.com/Listening_Room/preview.cfm?langid=1.

145 Hear at Home, downloadable guide: medel.com/us/rehabilitation/.

146 Cochlear Implant Online follows the CI industry; see cochlearimplantonline.com/site/2013-was-a-big-year-for-the-cochlear-implant-industry-whats-in-the-store-for-2014/.

147 sonitusmedical.com/product/soundbite-in-detail.cfm.

148 "Child Hears Sound in First FDA-Approved Clinical Trial of ABI in the U.S.," *Hearing Review*, August 4, 2014.

149 newsoffice.mit.edu/2014/cochlear-implants-with-no-exterior-hardware-0209.

150 physicsworld.com/cws/article/news/2014/feb/20/new-cochlear-implant-takes-the-middle-road.

151 Cochlear Implant Online: cochlearimplantonline.com/site/2013-was-a-big-year-for-the-cochlear-implant-industry-whats-in-the-store-for-2014/.

152 HLAA Cochlear Implants: hearingloss.org/content/cochlear-implants.

153 FDA: fda.gov/MedicalDevices/ProductsandMedicalProcedures/ImplantsandProsthetics/CochlearImplants/.

154 NIDCD: nidcd.nih.gov/staticresources/health/hearing/FactSheetCochlearImplant.pdf.

155 Johns Hopkins: hopkinsmedicine.org/otolaryngology/specialty_areas/listencenter/cochlear_info.html.

Part Five: Changing the Way We Think About Hearing Loss

Chapter 22, The Dangers of Denial and Ignorance

156 Sergei Kochkin of the Better Hearing Institute (BHI) says 95 percent of those with sensorineural hearing loss could benefit from hearing aids. Hi HealthInnovations says 90 percent of all with hearing loss could benefit.

157 Pichora-Fuller: 309.

158 *Hearing Review*, December 16, 2014.

159 For further discussion on the relationship between hearing loss and cognition, see "Hearing Loss Linked to Dementia." Katherine Griffin, aarp.org/health/brain-health/info-07-2013/hearing-loss-linked-to-dementia.html.

160 Improvement of Cognitive Function After Cochlear Implantation in Elderly Patients. archotol.jamanetwork.com/article.aspx?articleid=2195885.

Chapter 23, What We Can Do

161 Staab, hearinghealthmatters.org/waynesworld/2014/call-customers/.

ACKNOWLEDGMENTS

I owe thanks to dozens of people for their contributions to this book.

First, I would like to thank the readers of *Shouting Won't Help* and my blogs for writing to me with their own experiences and their own suggestions, many of which I have incorporated into this book. I've also learned a great deal from people who have attended my talks around the country. Their questions prompt new ideas and new areas of research. So thank you to all who have shared your experiences and broadened my understanding of hearing loss.

Many experts helped me with the more technical sections of the book: I want to specifically mention Cynthia Compton-Conley for her help with assistive listening devices, Juliette Sterkens for her help with induction looping, and Barbara Weinstein for her help sorting out what goes on at the audiologist's office and the tangled world of hearing aids.

Knowledgeable friends read many sections of the book, among them Richard Einhorn, Roy Kulick, Paul Lurie, Ed O'Brien, and David Baldridge. Drs. Darius Kohan and Anil Lalwani helped me with the chapter on cochlear implants. David Kirkwood and Holly Hosford-Dunn at Hearing Health & Technology Matters both read sections of the book and offered counsel on the hearing health industry. HHTM is one of my most reliable sources for news about developments in the hearing loss world.

I also owe thanks to Neil Bauman for allowing me to quote him so freely, and to the hilarious and smart Gael Hannan, who generously allowed me to reprint several long sections from her own weekly blog.

My fellow board members at the Hearing Loss Association of America have been an invaluable source of information for me. I particularly want to thank James Saunders, who as head of the nominating committee recruited me for the board, and Margaret Wallhagen for her insights into hearing loss and aging. Brenda Battat, the former executive director of HLAA, read the book in an early draft and offered insights gleaned from many years of experience with hearing loss and with HLAA.

Two people read the book thoroughly and more than once: Barbara Weinstein, professor and Founding Executive Officer of the Doctor of Audiology Program at the CUNY Graduate Center, and her student Jennifer Gilligan, soon to be Dr. Jennifer Gilligan. I owe them both immense thanks for their close reading and for their patience.

That's a lot of helpers for a single book. Nevertheless, errors may still have crept in and of course I take full responsibility for them. Since this is primarily an ebook, it's easy to correct mistakes, so please do point them out.

Much gratitude to my brilliant editor, Susan Bolotin, who has been the editorial director at Workman for as many years as I can remember and who has built it into one of the best publishing companies anywhere. I am so pleased to be a Workman author. The man- and woman-power brought to bear on this book has been mind-boggling. Specific mention must be made of Samantha O'Brien, whose many queries and observations were pretty much always on the mark. As a former editor myself, I know a good one when I see one, and Samantha is that. Janet Vicario came up with the boisterously engaging cover. Thanks to all at Workman, including Page Edmunds, Selina Meere, Randall Lotowycz, James Wehrle, Rebecca Schmidt, Thea James, Walter Weintz, David Schiller, Andrea Fleck-Nisbet, Jenny Lee, Moira Kerrigan, Beth Levy, Ariana Abud, Annie O'Donnell, Jacquelynne Hudson, and Linh Thoi.

My agent, Jim Levine, understood the need for this book right from the start, even while others wondered if I hadn't already written it. As it turned out, he was right: The two books complement each other but rarely overlap. Jim is the fastest email responder I know and the most soothing person in the world when one has an unseemly meltdown.

Finally, thanks again to my now adult children, Will Menaker (an editor himself) and Elizabeth Menaker (who always knows exactly what I'm trying to say, which is why she has become a psychologist). And gratitude, as always, to my husband, Dan, for his exacting literary standards and his unfailing encouragement. His patience and his sense of humor have helped us both through difficult times. Living with someone with hearing loss is not always easy, even if that person is me.

CPSIA information can be obtained
at www.ICGtesting.com
Printed in the USA
LVOW04s1734021216
515533LV00009B/446/P